Teen Self-Care

Editor: Tracy Biram

Volume 395

243392

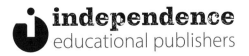

independence
educational publishers

First published by Independence Educational Publishers

The Studio, High Green

Great Shelford

Cambridge CB22 5EG

England

Copyright

Photocopy licence

ISBN-13: 978 1 86168 853 8

Printed in Great Britain

Zenith Print Group

Contents

Introduction

Teen Self-Care is Volume 395 in the **issues** series. The aim of the series is to offer current, diverse information about important issues in our world, from a UK perspective.

ABOUT TEEN SELF-CARE

Looking after yourself, both mentally and physically is very important. But we sometimes need to learn how to do this effectively. From mindfulness to vaccinations, we explore the best ways to look after ourselves and keep us healthy and happy.

OUR SOURCES

Titles in the **issues** series are designed to function as educational resource books, providing a balanced overview of a specific subject.

The information in our books is comprised of facts, articles and opinions from many different sources, including:

♦ Newspaper reports and opinion pieces

♦ Website factsheets

♦ Magazine and journal articles

♦ Statistics and surveys

♦ Government reports

♦ Literature from special interest groups.

A NOTE ON CRITICAL EVALUATION

Because the information reprinted here is from a number of different sources, readers should bear in mind the origin of the text and whether the source is likely to have a particular bias when presenting information (or when conducting their research). It is hoped that, as you read about the many aspects of the issues explored in this book, you will critically evaluate the information presented.

It is important that you decide whether you are being presented with facts or opinions. Does the writer give a biased or unbiased report? If an opinion is being expressed, do you agree with the writer? Is there potential bias to the 'facts' or statistics behind an article?

ASSIGNMENTS

In the back of this book, you will find a selection of assignments designed to help you engage with the articles you have been reading and to explore your own opinions. Some tasks will take longer than others and there is a mixture of design, writing and research-based activities that you can complete alone or in a group.

FURTHER RESEARCH

At the end of each article we have listed its source and a website that you can visit if you would like to conduct your own research. Please remember to critically evaluate any sources that you consult and consider whether the information you are viewing is accurate and unbiased.

Useful Websites

www.bda.uk.com

www.blurtitout.org

www.bma.org.uk

www.cancerresearchuk.org

www.dentalhealth.org

www.educatingmatters.co.uk

www.healthforteens.co.uk

www.independent.co.uk

www.jostrust.org.uk

www.metro.co.uk

www.nhs.uk

www.savethestudent.org

www.telegraph.co.uk

www.theconversation.com

www.topdoctors.co.uk

www.wearencs.com

www.youngpeopleshealth.org.uk

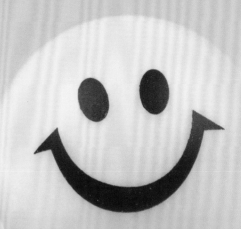

What is self-care?

Everyone is talking about self-care at the moment - but exactly what is it?

Basically, self-care is doing things to improve and preserve our mental and physical health. It's learning how to look after ourselves, so we can live in the happiest and healthiest way.

It can be something as simple as taking time to pamper yourself with a face-mask and bubble bath, to making sure you are up-to date with your vaccinations. Self-care can mean different things for different people, you need to find the right things for you, and it will be fun trying some different activities out!

Getting into the habit of self-care is important for teens as then it sets a precedent for looking after yourself for the rest of your life. It can also help with things such as exam stress and anxiety, and help to relieve some of the pressures from parents, school or friends.

Taking time out for yourself has so many positive benefits, it can help to improve our self-esteem and improve relationships. If we feel happier with ourselves then it makes it easier to reach our goals.

Some of the different activities that can help to calm you and give you a break from your worries could include: listening to music, cuddling a pet, going for a walk or watching a movie. Now, most of these things are free to do, meaning you don't need to spend a penny to give yourself a little happiness!

Why is self-care so important?

Well, learning about looking after your health and wellbeing will help to improve your life choices which, in turn, leads to better health, both mentally and physically.

If you know how to stay physically healthy, and care for things such as nutrition, hygiene, exercise etc. then you will be more likely to seek medical care if needed.

You will be able to tell if you aren't feeling as healthy as you should be, or if your mental health is suffering, and put in place changes and, if necessary, seek help from others.

What types of self-care are there?

Physical self-care is looking after your body by doing things such as:

♦ choosing healthy, nutritious food

♦ exercise

♦ hygiene

Emotional self-care is looking after your mind by doing things such as:

♦ giving your self a 'pep-talk'

♦ saying 'no' to things that cause stress

♦ pampering yourself

Spiritual self-care is looking after your soul by doing things such as:

♦ acts of kindness

♦ meditation

♦ spending time outside

Of course, you need to find your own routines and hobbies and the things listed above are just a guide. Choose things that you enjoy and make you feel happy. Some, you might already be doing without thinking about it, but if you think that you need more 'me time', make sure you make some time in your daily routine. Why not make a list of the self-care activities that you like and see where you can fit them in in your life.

Self-care vs. self-love: what's the difference?

Self-care and self-love are probably terms that we've heard before. But we might not know what they mean in practice. It can also be tricky to untangle self-care from self-love and to work out where one ends and the other begins.

What is self-care?

Self-care encompasses all the things we do to care for ourselves physically, emotionally, mentally and spiritually.

It can range from basic self-care, such as cleaning our teeth and going to bed at a reasonable time, to the things that help us feel better but aren't perhaps as essential, such as setting some time aside to read a book or treating ourselves to our favourite bubble bath.

What is self-love?

The dictionary definition of self-love is 'the instinct or desire to promote one's own well-being; regard for or love of one's self'.

Self-love is all about unconditionally accepting ourselves. It includes how we talk to ourselves, our feelings about ourselves, and some of our actions. It's not about thinking that every single part of our personality and body are fabulous. But it is about loving ourselves despite any perceived imperfections.

Misconceptions about self-care

When we talk about caring for ourselves physically, emotionally and mentally, we're talking about looking after ourselves, starting with our basic needs and working up. Our basic needs include feeling safe, secure and warm, taking our medication as prescribed, having adequate food and water, and getting enough rest.

Once we've covered our basic needs, we can think about things like creating healthy boundaries, managing our relationships, coping with money and bills, keeping our living space clean, being creative, learning, and working towards our full potential.

There's a misconception that self-care has to cost a fortune. Bath bombs, pampering sessions and spa days could all form part of our self-care. But self-care is much broader and will differ from person to person.

Misconceptions about self-love

Sometimes, when people are described as someone who 'loves themselves', it's in a negative context. There's a misconception that loving ourselves means we're boastful, self-important, and have an overly-inflated opinion of ourselves.

We use the term 'self-love' differently. When we use it, we're talking about wrapping ourselves in a hug. Caring for,

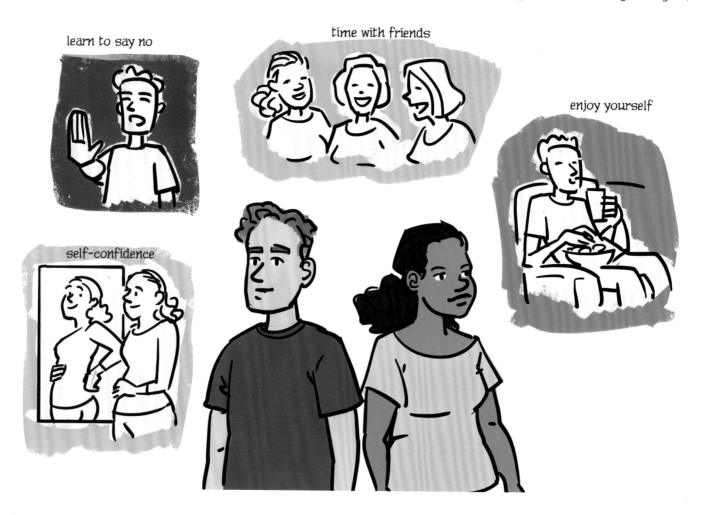

learn to say no

time with friends

enjoy yourself

self-confidence

2

and being kind to ourselves. Seeing ourselves as worthy; someone who deserves to be comfortable and okay.

We don't believe these things because we're egotistical, self-important or vain, but because we deserve to be loved, cared for, and okay.

'Nobody can love you until you love yourself'

There is a quote that pops up all over the place. There are multiple variations of it, but the general sentiment is the same; nobody can or will love us until we love ourselves.

This isn't true.

It's a damaging myth that many of us interpret as 'I don't love myself so nobody will ever love me'. If we think about it, most of us have at least one person, animal, or thing that we love despite not knowing where they fall on the 'self-love-o-meter'.

If we love someone who struggles with self-love, it can hurt to see them struggling with it because we care deeply about them. But it doesn't make us love them any less.

Can they be linked?

The short answer is yes.

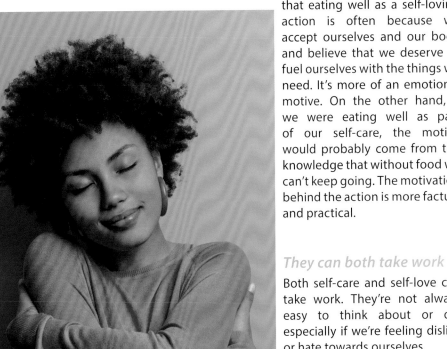

Self-care can help us to get to a point where we love ourselves. If we begin to prioritise self-care (however hard it may be), that can slowly help us to feel a little more 'human'. Self-care can teach us that actually, we do deserve to be cared for. We do deserve to be looked after. It can help us to gain a sense of self-respect and start to love who we are.

It can go the other way, too. When we start to love ourselves, our self-care often improves. Loving ourselves can help to reduce our levels of self-neglect. We might start to see our worth. To value ourselves and start doing things like going to the dentist for the first time in years.

Do we have to love ourselves to carry out self-care?

Self-love is not a prerequisite to self-care.

We can care for ourselves whether we love ourselves or not. Everybody goes through patches where self-love is tricky, but that doesn't mean that we need to stop caring for ourselves. It might be harder to keep up our self-care when we don't love ourselves, but it's not impossible.

How do they differ?

In general, self-love centres around the thoughts and feelings we have about ourselves whereas self-care focuses on our actions. That's not to say that we can't carry out acts of self-love or think about self-care. It's a general idea as opposed to a black and white concept.

If someone asked us how we were and we answered 'self-care' or 'care' it wouldn't make sense because it's not a feeling in the same way that 'love' is.

In contrast, if someone asked what we were up to and we said 'self-love', it would make less sense than if we said 'self-care'.

Some actions would class as both self-loving and self-caring actions, such as eating a balanced diet. The difference is that eating well as a self-loving action is often because we accept ourselves and our body and believe that we deserve to fuel ourselves with the things we need. It's more of an emotional motive. On the other hand, if we were eating well as part of our self-care, the motive would probably come from the knowledge that without food we can't keep going. The motivation behind the action is more factual and practical.

They can both take work

Both self-care and self-love can take work. They're not always easy to think about or do, especially if we're feeling dislike or hate towards ourselves.

Both of them are things that we can work on, though. We can learn to love ourselves and we can start small with self-care and slowly build it up. We don't have to do it alone, either, we can access support from our friends, family or professionals.

Wherever we stand on the self-care and self-love scale, it's important to remember that we're not alone. We're not the only one who feels as we do, and we won't feel this way forever.

'Self-care' is more than bubble baths

Looking after yourself can include mundane tasks such as hoovering your bedroom regularly – not exclusively glamorous holidays abroad and spa days.

By Marina Politis

The term 'self-care' has become a buzzword recently, featuring heavily in the dialogue surrounding mental health.

It is often a hashtag accompanied by pictures of luxurious bubble baths or sunsets, or a proclamation of having started a new hobby, be this jogging, yoga or crocheting.

Although the increased acknowledgement of the importance in taking time for ourselves and prioritising our wellbeing is a positive, the conversation surrounding self-care still has a way to go, and our narrative surrounding it is not always solely constructive.

This is not to say that we should neglect self-care – it should always be a priority – but we need to expand our definition of what self-care is and think critically about the motivations behind our perceived self-care.

Self-care shouldn't be a tool to mask what are underlying issues that need addressing. When does a glass of wine to destress at the end of a day become a negative coping strategy, that in fact embodies the opposite of what self-care is and only lets us be in denial of things that might be bothering us? When is a daily run no longer a healthy habit but in fact a form of disordered exercise?

This isn't to say we shouldn't treat ourselves with a glass of wine, takeaway or pint of ice cream, or burn off steam at the gym, but, these activities shouldn't solely be a form of escapism. Self-care has to mean reflecting on the sources of any stress, unhappiness or other negative emotions, and identifying methods to minimise these in the long term.

Self-care is also often promoted as an investment in the time that we can be productive. The elusive work-life balance is seen as an ideal where we ought to maximise the output in all aspects of our life. Can it be that self-care, however, contributes to this toxic notion of productivity?

Could the life element of the work-life equation not stand in isolation, without having to be a tool to maximise what we achieve in work or studies? We are told to sleep for eight hours because we will study better and nourish ourselves to optimise our concentration, but why not just do this for ourselves?

Sleeping well to feel rested and nourishing ourselves because our bodies and minds are worthy of care is enough of a reason. Self-care is not only justified where we see the results through increases in traditional measure of productivity

We must also ensure that the promotion of self-care doesn't shift the responsibility that decision- and policy-makers hold in needing to prioritise mental health, on to those who are themselves struggling. While strategies such as mindfulness

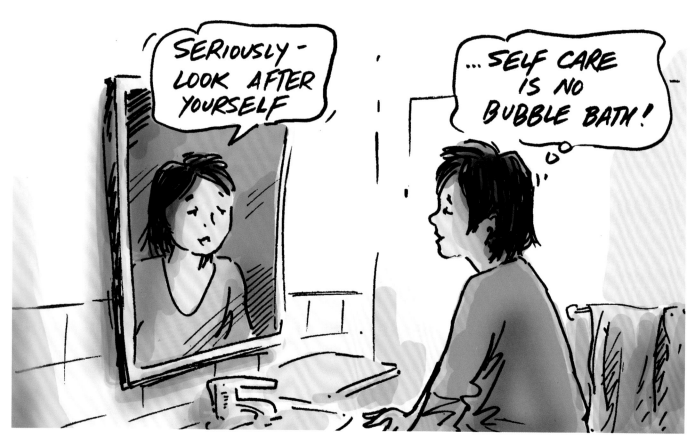

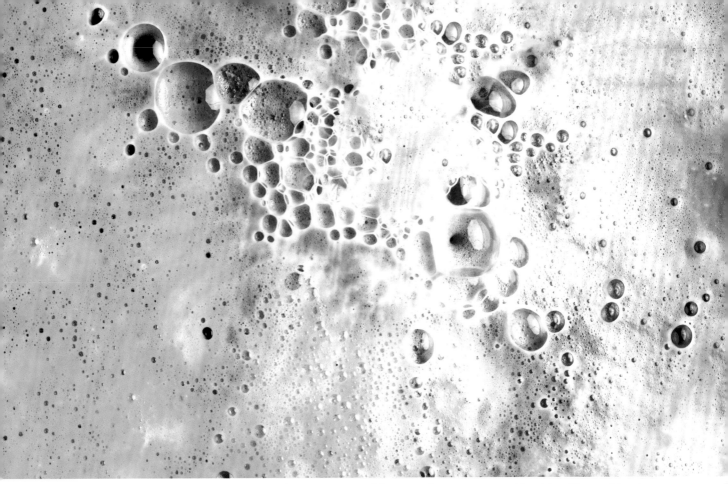

will no doubt be useful to many, they are not a solution to the UK's mental health crisis.

NHS mental health services, with their endlessly long waiting lists, need greater investment; universities must put further resources into counselling services that are at capacity, rather than therapy dogs and mandatory welfare lectures; and employers review their working conditions, rather than host staff yoga sessions. We need systemic change, not hollow sentiments asking individuals to look after themselves in a system that does not look after them.

In looking after ourselves as individuals, how do we include the 'less-glamorous' acts of self-care in the conversation surrounding mental health and wellbeing? When we talk about self-care only in terms of facemasks, cake and social connection, is this suggesting that those individuals who find that their mental health isn't managed by these acts, are not working hard enough at self-care or have somehow failed?

My self-care is a carefully concocted recipe of ensuring to set time aside for friends and family; getting outside and moving (often acquainting myself with squirrels in our local botanical garden) and spending time away from medicine. Just as important as this, however, is focusing on the basics of maintaining a healthy routine, with adequate sleep and regular meals.

Changing my sheets and hoovering my bedroom isn't interesting or exciting self-care, but it is important and we must challenge the notion that all self-care is 'instagramable' or pretty. For me, all of the aforementioned strategies are built up on the foundation of a daily antidepressant, and engaging in support and therapy, while staying accountable and honest about my mental health with my friends, even when I would rather just say that 'everything is fine'.

For those of us where self-care does mean taking medication each morning, making the time to go to therapy, or prioritising our wellbeing over other domains of our life, such as academics, it can still be difficult to justify this to the external world.

The antidepressant I pop out of its foil each morning does not make me a lesser medical student, or mean much at all – so why is this still harder to disclose than talking about a Sunday 'self-care' hike or brunch? We need to change the culture surrounding mental health in medicine by having open, honest conversations, and I hope that through blog posts like these, we can begin to change the dialogue surrounding mental health and reduce the stigma that still exists.

Self-care is unique to each individual and whether your self-care takes the form of a repeat prescription or a run; a bubble bath or a therapy session; learning to set boundaries and say 'no' or baking – all of these are valid. No one form of self-care trumps the other, and we need to talk about the full spectrum of what looking after our mental health can entail.

16 November 2020

Sometimes self-care is doing the things you don't want to do

By Tanyel Mustafa

What does self-care look like to you?

Instagram's answer is a bubble bath with candles lit and perfectly placed in the shot.

Sometimes, these things have their place in a self-care routine – a bath can serve to revitalise you and provide a moment of relief from stressful situations.

But we'd be duped if we believed that's the epitome of self-care or that self-care is always indulgent, luxurious, pleasant.

For some people seeing this bubblegum version of self-care is damaging and compromises their view on their own self-care rituals, which for someone in a particularly difficult mental state, might be as simple as getting dressed in the morning.

Suddenly, that looks subpar to a rose-petal-filled hot tub.

Often the biggest drivers of change in a person's life are born out of uncomfortable decisions, tough conversations, and actions that at first will cause upset.

As well as the pretty and aesthetically-pleasing side to self-care, there's the ugly side that's seldom spoken of.

That might include: saying 'no' to a loved one, leaving a relationship, and asserting boundaries.

Dr Roberta Babb, psychologist and co-founder of The Hanover Centre, tells Metro.co.uk: 'Self-care has unfortunately become synonymous with long baths, walks and other activities that people can find quite self-indulgent.

'Self-care is a much broader concept which essentially includes the practice of taking an active role in protecting your own wellbeing (emotional, physical, environmental and social), particularly during periods of stress.'

Being an active part of your wellbeing can mean doing things you don't want to do.

For Rina*, who recently changed her career, leaving her previous toxic job was a vital but anxiety-inducing experience.

She tells Metro.co.uk: 'I left the industry I had worked in for years because of the horrific way that they treated their staff.

'It was affecting my personal life – I was constantly living in fear of my boss who would make everything personal, tell me I was lucky to work there and yet they would continue to verbally abuse their staff.

'Leaving was a true act of self-care for both my mental and physical health, even if it meant starting over, and I haven't ever regretted that decision.'

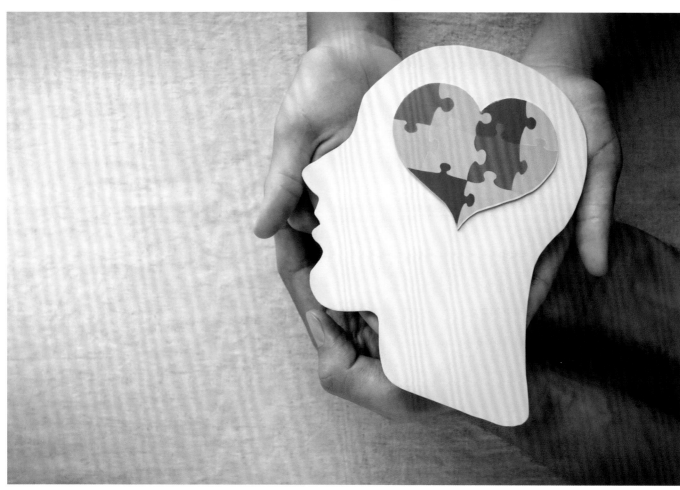

The initial discomfort Rina felt in making the decision ultimately was necessary in order to make a change that has benefitted her long-term. She is now happy in her new job.

Dr Babb believes there is a place for both kinds of self-care – the acts that are instantly soothing but don't promise to solve anything, and the acts that are incremental to creating a better future.

'They work to relieve different types of stress, and use different forms of energy to help you feel safe in your body, feelings, emotions, thoughts, environment and relationships,' she explains.

'However, the tricky thing can be recognising and deciding when to use behaviours that soothe you and when to use behaviours that actively change a situation.

'To help you identify when you should use particular self-care activities, it is important for you to understand your stress-response. This will help you identify a range of activities that you can use which work to manage the different areas of your stress response.

'Activities that soothe you primarily work to calm or reduce your level of emotional and physical arousal.

'Activities that actively change a situation work to create a space or separation between you and something else (such as a person, relationship, emotion, experience or event) which can relieve tension and stress.'

The key to maintaining adequate self-care is to have a 'variety of strategies', according to Dr Babb, so that means incorporating both styles.

When Scarlet was unhappy with her body, coupled with tackling mental health concerns, she knew she had to make changes that were initially painful.

It was hard enough for her to get out of bed to make time for the gym, but, she tells us: 'I had to run to the bathroom to cry the first few times because I didn't like what I saw in the mirror.

'It took a good month to feel comfortable again.'

Now beginning to feel better, that challenging first step laid the path to a habit that has benefitted her both mentally and physically.

As the old adage goes, sometimes it gets worse before it gets better.

While these acts may not typically look like self-care – due to the reality that they're not things we look forward to doing and there's the risk of opening emotional wounds – they are an important part of sustaining good mental health.

When we know it's time to get proactive about our self-care, it can be hard to do so – we may even want to put off doing certain things that we know will serve us later on.

'When we think of protection, one neglected strategy involves boundaries,' says Dr Babb.

'Recognising and asking for what you need (through identifying, communicating and reinforcing boundaries) is a form of self-care.

'These acts can become important elements of your growth and personal change, as they demonstrate the sense of

Dr Babb's guide to figuring out the kind of self-care you need to enact

Developing a 'five areas' formulation for yourself. This is a clear way to describe your own thoughts, feelings, behaviour and physiological response to external and internal events and how they may interact.

1. To do this first identify the things that stress you (external and internal to you).

2. Then identify the thoughts that these events trigger for you.

3. Then identify the emotions that you feel in response to the stressor(s).

4. Then identify any bodily sensations that you may experience when you are stressed.

5. Then identify the behaviours or things that you may do in response to the stress – both helpful and unhelpful.

This then allows you to examine your stress response and find a variety of strategies that may work for you.

integrity, compassion and respect you have for yourself.'

Whether you're setting boundaries with yourself or with others, it can be challenging.

Setting them alone means you have no one but yourself to hold accountable.

Setting them with others relies on them respecting your choices, and then, failing that, your ability to rethink your relationship with them.

Dr Babb says we often feel guilty for trying to assert ourselves in this way with other people, but she warns 'without boundaries you can become vulnerable to being overwhelmed and emotionally hurt'.

She advises, for those who struggle with this, to be clear and focused on your communication and to identify your talking points beforehand.

You should also consider what your desired outcome of the conversation is, what may happen if you don't get that, and what you realistically cannot control.

Self-care is by no means a simple thing, but it would be foolish to assume that it will always feel instantly good.

Self-care isn't equivalent to having fun.

Sometimes you've got to create space to heal first.

Name has been changed to protect the person's identity

13 May 2021

Key data on young people

An extract.

Health promotion and use of health services

Over 80% of secondary school pupils in the UK receive teenage vaccinations including MMR, MenACWY and HPV

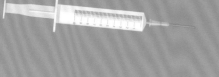

46% of 15 year olds have decay in their permanent teeth

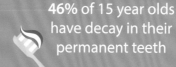

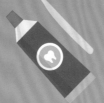

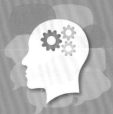

The number of referrals to specialist children's mental health services has **increased by 26%** over the last five years.

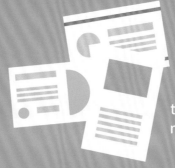

For every 1000 people under 18, although approximately 140 will have mental health problems, **only 18** will be on the formal child and adolescent mental health services caseload

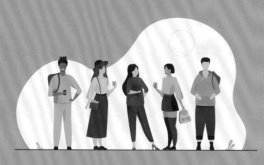

Schools, parents, peers and the voluntary sector all play a major part in health promotion for young people

52% of boys and 57% of girls in Year 10 (aged 14-15) have visited their GP in the past 3 months

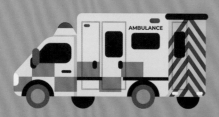

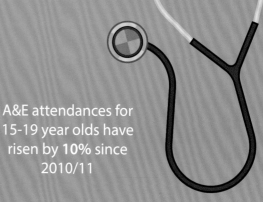

A&E attendances for 15-19 year olds have risen by **10%** since 2010/11

A third (32%) of those age 16-25 who could not get to see the GP when they wanted then went to Accident and Emergency

Source: AYPH | Key Data on Young People 2019

Health promotion

One of the key challenges for young people is the transition to independence that takes place across the second decade of life. Learning how to recognise health issues and manage the process of getting help is very important at this time. Supporting young people through this process means empowering them to take control of their health and giving them the information they need to seek appropriate services.

Health promotion for this age group tends to focus on sexual health, physical activity, smoking, drinking and drug use, and diet and nutrition. Interventions to promote health can address individual behaviour and can also target wider social and environmental factors. Interventions aimed at changing individual behaviour include stopping smoking programmes, promotion of dental checkups, or school based relationship and sex education. Wider population interventions might include media information campaigns or policy such as advertising bans, tax incentives and pricing structures (for example, in relation to alcohol sales) and clearer food labelling. There are very few representative data on how these wider population interventions might impact on young people, mainly because undertaking the studies that would answer the question is methodologically complex and expensive, and the effect sizes are probably small at the individual level. However, we do have more information on the effectiveness of health promotion as delivered through schools, vaccination programmes, access to helplines and individual level support and advice.

When asked about sources of helpful information, for example about drug use, young people report that they use a wide range of sources. Questions asked in the 2013 HSCIC Smoking, Drinking and Drug Use Survey (SDDU) showed teachers and parents came top of the list. The findings were similar to those in the 2012 National Survey on Sexual Attitudes and Lifestyle (Natsal-3), showing schools, parents and health professionals were the preferred sources for information about sex and relationships for 16-24 year olds.

Chart 8.2 draws on data from the Exeter Schools Health Education Unit to show peers feature strongly as sources of information and support among 12-15 year olds. However, many young people often report turning first to their family for information, help and advice, with the exception of sex and relationships and parental conflict. These findings illustrate the value of providing support to parents in communicating with their teenage children. Importantly, primary care services also feature as a source of advice and help for a wide range of issues, highlighting the value of helping GPs and others to understand and prioritise young people's health.

Chart 8.2: Where 12-15 year olds first go for help or information about emotional and physical health issues,England, 2014

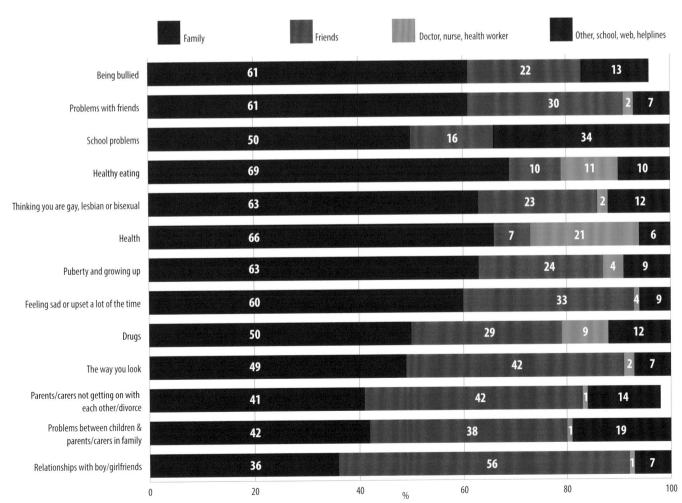

Source: Balding and Regis (2014), Young People into 2014

As these surveys show, schools clearly play a major role in health promotion through the provision of personal, social, health and economic education (PSHE). The wider aim of PSHE is '…to equip pupils with a sound understanding of risk and with the knowledge and skills necessary to make safe and informed decisions'. The 2017 Child and Social Work Act made sex, relationships and health education statutory in all secondary schools in England from September 2020. It will be important to watch how this is applied in practice, and to measure what young people think about the information they are given. There is also increasing evidence for modifying the whole school environment as an intervention to reduce bullying victimisation in schools, and to address closely related risk and health outcomes in young people. Whole school approaches or interventions are multi-faceted and encourage the active participation of parents, students, teachers and the wider school community, to plan, implement and evaluate school policies, procedures, teaching and learning and professional development.

An important part of the landscape of health promotion and early intervention relates to youth service provision. This includes community based universal and early intervention, some school based early interventions, support for vulnerable young people, and other services. A number of local authorities no longer provide some or all of these services.

Immunisation

In the UK the human papillomavirus (HPV) vaccine has been routinely offered to girls aged 12-13 since 2008, and this is due to be extended to boys from September 2019. It helps protect against cancers caused by HPV, including cervical cancer, some mouth and throat cancers, some cancers of the anal and genital areas, and genital warts. Recent analysis from Scotland has concluded that the programme has led to an 89% reduction in preinvasive cervical disease.

> Routine human papillomavirus (HPV) vaccination of girls in Scotland aged 12-13 has led to an **89% reduction** in preinvasive cervical disease
>
> Source: Palmer et al (2019)

In 2017/18, 83.4% of Year 9 females in England completed the two-dose HPV vaccination course. The uptake is similar in other UK countries, at 83% in Wales in 2018, for example. Data from England have shown that the prevalence of high-risk HPV has reduced with the increasing number of young women who receive the vaccine.

Secondary school age children are also due a teenage booster of the measles, mumps and rubella (MMR) vaccination, and a dose of the MenACWY vaccine, which protects against serious infections including meningitis and septicaemia. The MenACWY vaccine was added to the national immunisation programme in August 2015, and can be requested from the GP up until the young person's 25th birthday. It is advised that students going to university for the first time ensu that they have had their dose. The average coverage for th school based MenACWY adolescent vaccination programm in England in 2018 was 84.6%.

Dental health

In 2016 Public Health England launched the Children's Or Health Improvement Programme Board, with the aim reductions in the number of children with tooth decay and reduction in the oral health gap for disadvantaged familie

However there has not been a Children's Dental Healt Survey since 2013. At that time a third of 12 year olds (24%) and nearly half of 15 year olds (46%) had decay in their permanent teeth. More than a quarter of 15 year olds reported being embarrassed to smile or laugh due to the condition of their teeth. Young people who were eligible for free school meals were twice as likely to have severe or extensive tooth decay.

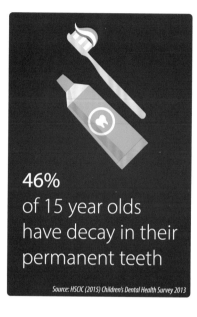

46% of 15 year olds have decay in their permanent teeth

Source: HSCIC (2015) Children's Dental Health Survey 2013

The most recent Adult Dental Health survey was undertaken even longe ago, in 2009, covering England, Wales and Northern Irelanc At that time only 23% of 16-24 year olds achieved 'excellen oral health', which included criteria such as having 21 o more natural teeth, 18 or more sound and untreated teet and roots and no decay detected at any site. In 1978 16 t 24 year olds had 27.4 teeth on average compared with 28. in 2009.

2019

www.youngpeopleshealth.org.uk

Why vaccination is safe and important

Vaccines are the most effective way to prevent infectious diseases. This page explains how vaccines work, what they contain and the most common side effects.

Be aware of anti-vaccine stories

Anti-vaccine stories are often spread online through social media.

They may not be based on scientific evidence and could put your child at risk of a serious illness.

Things you need to know about vaccines

Vaccines:

Do

✓ protect you and your child from many serious and potentially deadly diseases

✓ protect other people in your community – by helping to stop diseases spreading to people who cannot have vaccines

✓ undergo rigorous safety testing before being introduced – they're also constantly monitored for side effects after being introduced

✓ sometimes cause mild side effects that will not last long – some children may feel a bit unwell and have a sore arm for 2 or 3 days

✓ reduce or even get rid of some diseases – if enough people are vaccinated

Don't

✗ do not cause autism – studies have found no evidence of a link between the MMR vaccine and autism

✗ do not overload or weaken the immune system – it's safe to give children several vaccines at a time and this reduces the amount of injections they need

✗ do not cause allergies or any other conditions – all the current evidence tells us that vaccinating is safer than not vaccinating

✗ do not contain mercury (thiomersal)

✗ do not contain any ingredients that cause harm in such small amounts – but speak to your doctor if you have any known allergies such as eggs or gelatine

Why vaccines are important

Vaccination is the most important thing we can do to protect ourselves and our children against ill health. They prevent up to 3 million deaths worldwide every year.

Since vaccines were introduced in the UK, diseases like smallpox, polio and tetanus that used to kill or disable millions of people are either gone or seen very rarely.

Other diseases like measles and diphtheria have been reduced by up to 99.9% since their vaccines were introduced.

However, if people stop having vaccines, it's possible for infectious diseases to quickly spread again.

The World Health Organization (WHO) has listed vaccine hesitancy as one of the biggest threats to global health.

Vaccine hesitancy is where people with access to vaccines delay or refuse vaccination.

Measles and mumps in England

Measles and mumps are starting to appear again in England, even though the MMR vaccine is safe and protects against both diseases.

Measles and mumps cases have nearly doubled in recent years:

Measles and mumps cases in England

Year	Measles	Mumps
2016	530	573
2018	970	1061

This is serious as measles can lead to life-threatening complications like meningitis, and mumps can cause hearing loss.

Important

If 95% of children receive the MMR vaccine, it's possible to get rid of measles.

However, measles, mumps and rubella can quickly spread again if fewer than 90% of people are vaccinated.

How vaccines work

Vaccines teach your immune system how to create antibodies that protect you from diseases.

It's much safer for your immune system to learn this through vaccination than by catching the diseases and treating them.

Once your immune system knows how to fight a disease, it can often protect you for many years.

Herd immunity

Having a vaccine also benefits your whole community through 'herd immunity'.

If enough people are vaccinated, it's harder for the disease to spread to those people who cannot have vaccines. For example, people who are ill or have a weakened immune system.

Why vaccines are safe

All vaccines are thoroughly tested to make sure they will not harm you or your child.

It often takes many years for a vaccine to make it through the trials and tests it needs to pass for approval.

Once a vaccine is being used in the UK it's also monitored for any rare side effects by the Medicines and Healthcare products Regulatory Agency (MHRA).

Anyone can report a suspected side effect of vaccination to the MHRA through the Yellow Card Scheme.

Who cannot have vaccines

There are very few people who cannot have vaccines.

Generally, vaccines are only not suitable for:

- people who've had a serious allergic reaction (anaphylaxis) to a previous dose of the vaccine
- people who've had a serious allergic reaction to ingredients in the vaccine

People with weakened immune systems (for example, because of cancer treatment or a health condition) may also not be able to have some vaccines.

If you're not sure if you or your child can be vaccinated, check with a GP, practice nurse, health visitor or pharmacist.

Side effects of vaccination

Most of the side effects of vaccination are mild and do not last long.

The most common side effects of vaccination include:

- the area where the needle goes in looking red, swollen and feeling a bit sore for 2 to 3 days
- babies or young children feeling a bit unwell or developing a high temperature for 1 or 2 days

Some children might also cry and be upset immediately after the injection. This is normal and they should feel better after a cuddle.

Allergic reactions

It's rare for anyone to have a serious allergic reaction to a vaccination. If this does happen, it usually happens within minutes.

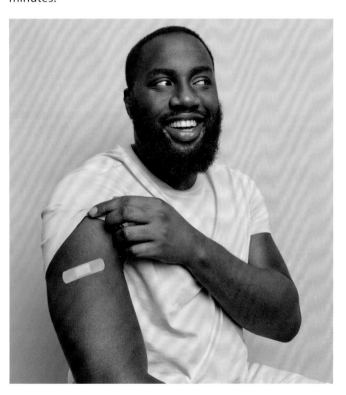

What's the difference between a live or killed vaccine?

Live (weakened) vaccines	Killed (destroyed) vaccines
Contain viruses or bacteria that have been weakened	Contain viruses or bacteria that have been destroyed
Cannot be given to people with a weakened immune system	Can still be given to people with a weakened immune system
Gives long-term protection	Often needs several doses or a booster vaccine for full protection

The person who vaccinates you or your child will be trained to deal with allergic reactions and treat them immediately. With prompt treatment, you or your child will make a good recovery.

Non-urgent advice: Speak to your GP or practice nurse if:

- you're worried about you or your child having a vaccine
- you're not sure if you or your child can have a vaccine

You could also ask a health visitor any questions you have about vaccines.

What's in a vaccine?

Most people are not concerned about vaccine ingredients and know that they are safe.

The main ingredient of any vaccine is a small amount of bacteria, virus or toxin that's been weakened or destroyed in a laboratory first.

This means there's no risk of healthy people catching a disease from a vaccine. It's also why you might see vaccines being called 'live' or 'killed' vaccines.

30 July 2019

Immunisation in secondary school: just the facts

In the UK we have one of the most successful immunisation programmes in the world.

This means that dangerous diseases, such as polio, diphtheria or tuberculosis, have pretty much disappeared in the UK.

But, these diseases could come back into the UK – if we stop vaccinating. These diseases are still around in many countries throughout the world, which is why it's so important to make sure you're protected!

What, where, when, who?

The following immunisations are offered in school, and are no longer available at your GP surgery:

In Year 8, from September 2019, both girls and boys will be offered 2 doses of the human papillomavirus (HPV) vaccination. The 2 doses are given from 6 months apart. If you're absent on the day the vaccine is given in school, don't worry as the immunisation team will make sure they see you at another time.

Additionally, in Year 8, if you didn't receive two doses of the measles, mumps and rubella (MMR) vaccine when you were younger, you will also be offered a single dose of MMR at the same time as your HPV vaccination. This is because there has been a significant rise in the number of cases of measles in recent years.

In Year 9, both girls and boys will be given two immunisations:

♦ Teenage booster – which protects against tetanus, diphtheria and polio

♦ Meningitis booster – which protects against A, C, W and Y strains of meningitis

Due to concerns about the impact of the Flu virus and COVID-19 co-circulating this year, from September 2020, all students in Year 7 will be offered the nasal flu vaccine in school.

It is vital that all those who are eligible get vaccinated in order to protect themselves, their families and the wider community. Young people, not in Year 7, who have underlying health conditions, will still be offered the flu vaccine by their GP.

The gelatine used in the manufacture of the nasal flu vaccine is not acceptable for some parents, therefore, for this flu season, parents will be able to opt for a gelatine-free injection instead. When making a decision to opt for the injectable vaccine, it's important to be aware that the gelatine-free injection:

1. Is less effective than the nasal flu
2. An injection into the muscle at the top of the arm can be uncomfortable; therefore your presence may be required
3. The injectable vaccine will be available later in the flu season and is dependent on stock levels. This means there may be a delay receiving it

The immunisations are given in school by healthcare professionals (nurses) who are very experienced at giving injections. Both injections are usually given one after the other, into the muscle at the top of your arm. It's usual for them to be given into the opposite arm to the one you write with. This is because your arm may feel a little achy afterwards and the nurses don't want to stop you from continuing with your school work!

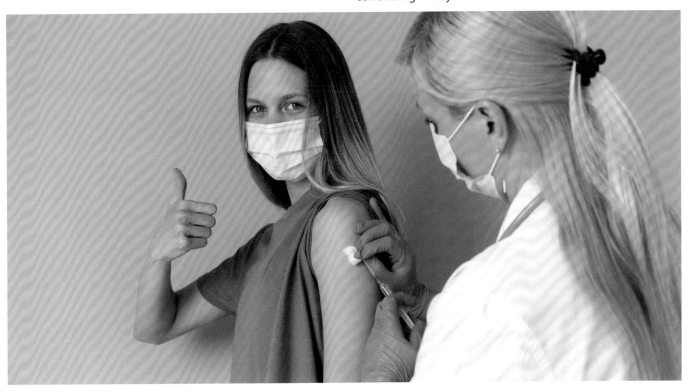

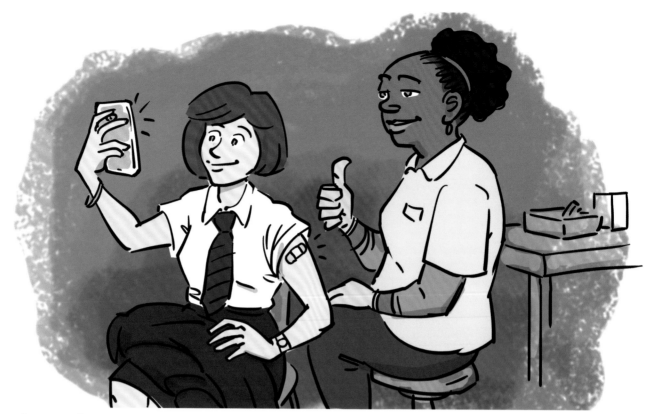

Depending on where you live you and your vaccination history, your parents will either receive information about how to give consent via email or text from school, or via a letter sent to your home address.

Some people get a headache and have general muscle aches for a day or two following your immunisations. These are very normal reactions to vaccinations and nothing to worry about. Let your parent or carer know if you do feel unwell and make sure you eat and drink well on the day of vaccinations.

Questions, questions

Before you have your immunisation, the health care professional will ask you some questions. For example:

♦ Are you feeling well today?

♦ Are you taking any medicines?

♦ Have you had any recent immunisations?

♦ Have you had a bad reaction to any immunisations in the past?

♦ Do you have any allergies?

♦ Do you have a bleeding disorder? (When you cut or bump yourself, if you bleed or bruise really badly we would like to know about it)

♦ Are you receiving treatment at a hospital or from a doctor?

We would also need to know if anyone is pregnant or thinks they could be pregnant. This is important for us to know, and can be discussed with the nurse in private.

How will I feel after the immunisation?

You may have a sore, red arm – this is normal and nothing to worry about. It's important to keep your arm moving as normal and carry on with your day.

It's common to have a headache, raised temperature or achy joints for a couple of days after the immunisation. It could be the body's natural response, or you could just have caught a different virus.

It's very important to drink plenty of fluids, such as water, to keep your body hydrated. You may wish to take a dose of paracetamol or ibuprofen. Please discuss this with an adult first and always follow the instructions on the packaging of these medications.

More serious side effects are very rare. The vaccines used meet rigorous safety standards to be licensed for the UK Immunisation Programme.

Consent

It's best and really great if you share the information about the immunisation with your parent/carer and complete the consent form together.

It's ok to make the decision yourself, but make sure you have all of the information and talk to the immunisation nurse on the day who will answer any questions you might have.

If you don't have your parent or carer's consent, it doesn't mean you can't have the immunisation. The immunisation nurse will to talk to you to make sure it's safe.

1 September 2020

Why it makes medical – and mathematical – sense to finally vaccinate boys against the HPV virus

An article from *The Conversation*.

THE C⊖NVERSATION

By Christian Yates, Senior Lecturer in Mathematical Biology, University of Bath

From September 2019, boys aged 12 and 13 in the UK are being offered free vaccination against the Human Papillomavirus (HPV) for the first time. HPV causes cervical cancer, and girls and young women have been receiving the vaccine for over ten years. So why is it being rolled out for boys too? And why only now?

One reason for giving the vaccine to boys is that the vast majority of cases of cervical cancer-causing HPV infections are transmitted through sexual intercourse. Men can carry the virus without symptoms and pass it on to their sexual partners.

In fact, HPV is the most frequently sexually transmitted disease in the world, and over 60% of all cervical cancers are caused by two HPV strains. Cervical cancer itself is the fourth most common cancer in women, with around half a million new cases and over quarter of a million deaths reported worldwide each year.

Unsurprisingly, given this high prevalence, when the first vaccines against HPV were approved in the US in 2006, there was great hope surrounding their potential. Mathematical modelling studies carried out around that time indicated that the most cost effective strategy would be to immunise adolescent girls between the ages of 12 and 13 – the likely future sufferers of cervical cancer.

But, as I uncover in my new book *The Maths of Life and Death* (along with many other surprising occasions where maths has played a crucial, but sometimes unseen, role) the mathematical models didn't capture the whole picture. Most of the analyses did not include an important feature of HPV in their assumptions: that the strains of HPV guarded against by the vaccine can also cause a range of non-cervical diseases in both women and men.

In July of 2018, a new mathematical study led to a recommendation that all boys in the UK be given the HPV vaccination at the same age as girls.

This is in part because as well as causing cervical cancer, HPV types 16 and 18 contribute to 50% of penile cancers, 80% of anal cancers, 20% of mouth, and 30% of throat cancers. In both the US and the UK, the majority of cancers caused by HPV are not cervical.

This fact came to the fore when the actor Michael Douglas was asked, during his recovery from throat cancer, if he regretted his lifetime of smoking and drinking. The actor candidly replied that he had no regrets about this, because his cancer had been caused by HPV, which he contracted through oral sex.

Warts and verrucas are also caused by different types of HPV, and 80% of people in the UK will be infected with one strain of HPV at some point during their lives.

So cervical cancer is an important part of the HPV picture, but it is not, by any means, the whole story. It seemed that the link to other cancers and diseases had been underestimated.

The rest of the picture

The public, perhaps aware only of HPV's role in cervical cancer, seemed to accept the decision to only vaccinate females. Why would we waste money vaccinating boys if they don't suffer from the headline HPV cancer?

On top of this, mathematical models into the impact of HPV vaccination suggested that by vaccinating a sufficiently high proportion of females, the prevalence of HPV-related diseases in males would also decline.

But imagine the outrage if a vaccination for human immunodeficiency virus (HIV) was given only to women for free, in the hope that men would be protected through women's immunity.

Perhaps the first point that critics would make (aside from the issues of partial vaccination coverage and vaccine inefficiency) would be about the protection of gay men – why should they be left defenceless against one of the most deadly viruses of our time, just because they don't have sex with women?

Exactly the same argument holds true in the case of HPV. Early mathematical studies had ignored the impact of same sex couplings on the dynamics of HPV spread.

Models that include homosexual relationships suggest a higher rate of sexual disease transmission than those which consider only heterosexual relationships. And the prevalence of HPV in men who have sex with men is significantly higher than in the general population.

When models were recalibrated to take into account homosexual relationships, protection afforded against non-cervical cancers, and new information on the length of protection that the HPV vaccination provides, it was found that vaccinating boys as well as girls became a more cost-effective option.

Now that the vaccination is finally here, available to boys as well as girls – in a move which will reduce the rates of many kinds of cancer as well as other HPV-related diseases.

This is good news for all of us. And on a personal note I am delighted that my son, as well as my daughter, will now be afforded equal protection against catching and spreading the virus that killed their grandmother. In the case of cervical cancer, as with many of the other cases I have investigated, maths really can be a matter of life and death.

27 September 2019

About cervical screening

What is cervical screening?

Cervical screening is a free health test available on the NHS as part of the national cervical screening programme. It helps prevent cervical cancer by checking for a virus called high-risk HPV and cervical cell changes. It is not a test for cancer.

It is your choice whether to go for cervical screening. We hope this information helps you make the best decision for you and your health.

If you have symptoms, contact your GP surgery about having an examination. Cervical screening is not for people who have symptoms.

Who is invited for cervical screening?

You should be invited for cervical screening if you have a cervix. Women are usually born with a cervix. Trans men, non-binary and intersex people may also have one.

In the UK, you are automatically invited for cervical screening if you are:

- between the ages of 25 to 64
- registered as female with a GP surgery.

You may get your first invite up to 6 months before you turn 25. You can book an appointment as soon as you get the invite.

How often will I be invited for cervical screening?

Your cervical screening result will help decide when you are next invited for cervical screening.

You may be invited:

- every year
- every 3 years
- every 5 years
- straight to colposcopy for more tests.

What are the benefits and risks of cervical screening?

You are invited for cervical screening because evidence shows that the benefits of the test outweigh any risks. Along with the HPV vaccine, cervical screening is the best way to protect against cervical cancer and prevents over 7 in 10 diagnoses. However, like any screening test, cervical screening is not perfect and there are some risks.

Benefits of cervical screening

Cervical screening aims to identify whether you are at higher risk of developing cervical cell changes or cervical cancer. This means you can get any care or treatment you need early.

England, Scotland and Wales now use HPV primary screening, which is even better as it is based on your individual risk. This means how frequently you are invited for cervical screening is based on your last result and within a timeframe that is safe for you.

Possible risks of cervical screening

In a few cases, cervical screening will give an incorrect result. This means it may say someone does not have HPV or cell changes when they do (a false negative). Going for cervical screening when invited can help reduce this risk, as it is likely HPV or cell changes that were missed would be picked up by the next test. It also means a result may say someone does have HPV or cell changes when they don't (a false positive), which could mean they are invited for tests or treatment they don't need.

Sometimes cell changes go back to normal without needing treatment. At the moment, we can't tell which cell changes will go back to normal, so treating means we can be sure we are preventing them from developing into cervical cancer. This means some people may have unnecessary treatment, which is called overdiagnosis or overtreatment. Using HPV primary screening should help prevent this.

It is hard to know exactly how many people are affected by these risks. But we do know, for those aged 25 to 64, the benefits of cervical screening outweigh the risks and most results will be clear.

Opting out of cervical screening

If you decide not have cervical screening, ask your GP to be taken off their invite list. If you change your mind, you can ask your GP to add you back to the list at any time.

Jo's Cervical Cancer Trust is an independent charity and cannot opt you out of the National Cervical Screening Programme.

Cervical screening FAQs

What is the difference between cervical screening and a smear test?

There is no difference between cervical screening and a smear test. They are two different names for the same test.

A smear test is the older name for the test. It was called that because of the way the test used to be done – cells were smeared on a glass slide, which was sent to the laboratory for testing.

The test is different now and most healthcare professionals call it cervical screening. Your letter will invite you to attend cervical screening, which is why we call it that in our information.

Why can't I have cervical screening unless I am age 25 to 64?

It is very rare to develop cervical cancer under the age of 25. It is also rare to develop cervical cancer over the age of 64, if you have had regular cervical screening.

How do I check for cancer?

- It's good to be aware of how your body usually looks and feels, but there's no need to check yourself at a set time or in a set way

- Take charge and speak to your doctor if you notice anything's that's not normal for you

- Spotting cancer at an early stage can save lives

This article explains our evidence-based views on self-checking for cancer. We know that this information may be surprising for some people. But the best research shows that there's no special time or way that you need to check your body.

We cover breasts or chest, and testicles in more detail on this page because these are the most talked about body parts when it comes to self-checking.

What should I look for?

You know your body best. If you notice anything that's unusual for you, or won't go away, make an appointment to speak to your doctor.

It's not possible to know all the different signs and symptoms of cancer, and it's not your job to know what's wrong. So the best thing you can do is to tell your doctor if you notice anything that's not normal for you. In most cases it won't be cancer – but if it is, spotting it early can make a real difference.

Symptoms that are difficult to see or touch

Some common cancer symptoms are easy to see. But others can happen inside your body or be a change to how your body works. These changes can be more difficult to spot or describe. But being aware of how you usually feel can help you notice when something's different.

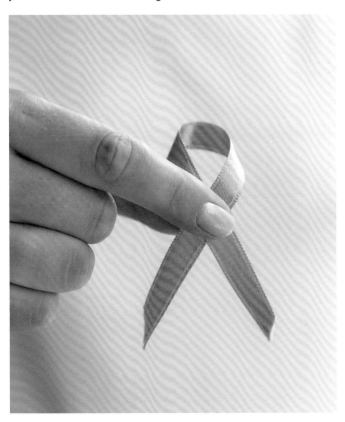

It might be a cough that lasts for a few weeks, a change in your poo, heartburn that keeps coming back or any other change that isn't normal for you. But whatever the symptom is, when something doesn't feel quite right – don't ignore it. Take charge and speak to your doctor.

And it's important not to put any unusual changes, aches or pains down to 'just getting older' or assume something is part of another health condition. If it's not normal for you, get it checked out.

How do I self-check for cancer?

Lots of people talk about doing 'self-checks' (also known as self-examinations or self-exams), to try and spot cancer early.

It's good to be aware of what your body is normally like, so it's easier to notice if anything changes. But there's no good evidence to suggest that regularly self-checking any part of your body in a set time or set way is helpful. It can actually do more harm than good, by picking up things which wouldn't have gone on to cause you problems.

Should I check my breasts or chest?

It is good to be breast aware. This means getting to know what your breasts or chest usually look and feel like, so you know what's normal for you. This includes knowing what your breasts are like at different times of the month.

But there is no need to worry about regularly checking your breasts or chest at a set time or in a set way. Research has shown that women who regularly self-check their breasts aren't any less likely to die from breast cancer. But they are almost twice as likely to have an unnecessary test (biopsy) on a lump that turns out not to be cancer.

Remember, it's still important to listen to your body and tell your doctor if you've noticed any unusual lumps or other changes that aren't normal for you. Whether it's your breasts, nipples or any other body part, if something's not quite right (no matter how you find it), get it checked out.

You can read more about breast changes to look out for on our signs and symptoms page.

Should I check my testicles?

It's a good idea to know what your testicles usually look and feel like, and to be aware of their normal size and weight. This can make it easier to spot unusual changes, which you should always let your doctor know about.

But there's no need to worry about regularly self-checking at a set time or in a set way. There is no specific self-checking method that has overall proven benefits.

21 October 2020

Signs and symptoms of cancer

This page covers some of the key signs and symptoms of cancer, including those which can be early signs. Not every person with cancer has symptoms. But spotting cancer early saves lives, so tell your doctor if you notice anything that isn't normal for you.

Keep reading below for more detailed information on the key cancer signs and symptoms. We have separate information on specific cancer types and their possible symptoms.

How do you know if you have cancer?

There are over 200 different types of cancer that can cause many different symptoms. Sometimes symptoms are linked to certain cancer types. But signs can also be more general, including weight loss, tiredness (fatigue) or unexplained pain.

You don't need to try and remember all the signs and symptoms of cancer, but we have listed some key ones to give you an idea of the kind of things to be aware of. These symptoms are more often a sign of something far less serious – but if it is cancer, spotting it early can make a real difference.

Remember, anyone can develop cancer, but it's more common as we get older. Most cases are in people aged 50 or over. Whatever your age, it's always best to listen to your body and talk to your doctor if something doesn't feel quite right. Whether it's a change that's new, unusual, or something that won't go away – get it checked out.

Cancer symptoms can be specific to a certain type of cancer or more general. Knowing the early signs of cancer can help identify whether you may have cancer sooner.

Some possible signs of cancer – like a lump – are better known than others. But just because some symptoms are more well known, doesn't mean they're more important, or more likely to be cancer. If you spot anything that isn't normal for you – don't ignore it. Whether it's on this list or not, get it checked out.

General cancer symptoms

Unexplained pain or ache

Pain is one way our bodies tell us that something is wrong. As we get older, it's more common to experience aches and pains. But unexplained pain could be a sign of something more serious.

Very heavy night sweats

Sweating at night can be caused by infections or it can be a side effect of certain medications. It's also often experienced by women around the time of the menopause. But very heavy, drenching night sweats can also be a sign of cancer.

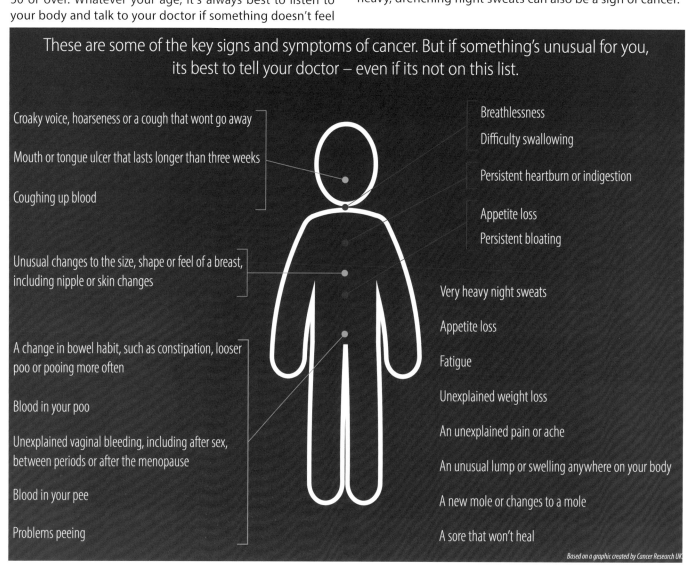

These are some of the key signs and symptoms of cancer. But if something's unusual for you, its best to tell your doctor – even if its not on this list.

Croaky voice, hoarseness or a cough that wont go away

Mouth or tongue ulcer that lasts longer than three weeks

Coughing up blood

Unusual changes to the size, shape or feel of a breast, including nipple or skin changes

A change in bowel habit, such as constipation, looser poo or pooing more often

Blood in your poo

Unexplained vaginal bleeding, including after sex, between periods or after the menopause

Blood in your pee

Problems peeing

Breathlessness

Difficulty swallowing

Persistent heartburn or indigestion

Appetite loss

Persistent bloating

Very heavy night sweats

Appetite loss

Fatigue

Unexplained weight loss

An unexplained pain or ache

An unusual lump or swelling anywhere on your body

A new mole or changes to a mole

A sore that won't heal

Based on a graphic created by Cancer Research UK

Unexplained weight loss

Small weight changes over time are quite normal, but if you lose a noticeable amount of weight without trying to, tell your doctor.

Unusual lump or swelling anywhere

Persistent lumps or swelling in any part of your body should be taken seriously. That includes any lumps in the neck, armpit, stomach, groin, chest, breast or testicle.

Fatigue

There are lots of reasons you may feel more tired than usual, particularly if you're going through a stressful event, or having troubles sleeping. But if you're feeling tired for no clear reason, it could be a sign that something is wrong - speak to your doctor.

Skin changes
Sore that won't heal

The skin repairs itself very quickly and any damage usually heals within a week or so. When a spot, wart or sore doesn't heal, even if it's painless, a doctor needs to check it.

New mole or changes to a mole

Most moles are harmless. But be aware of any new moles or existing moles that change in size, shape or colour, become crusty, itch, hurt, bleed or ooze. The ABCDE checklist gives more details about the key changes you should always tell your doctor about.

Other skin changes

Any unusual change in a patch of skin or a nail, whether it's a new change or has been there for a while, should be checked out by your doctor.

Symptoms that affect eating
Difficulty swallowing

Some medical conditions can make it difficult to swallow. Talk to your doctor if you are having difficulty swallowing and the problem doesn't go away.

Unusual heartburn or indigestion

It is normal to feel slight discomfort or pain sometimes after eating a large, fatty or spicy meal. But if you have heartburn (acid reflux) or indigestion a lot, or if it is particularly painful, then you should see your doctor.

Appetite loss

Appetite loss can happen for many different reasons. Speak to your doctor if you've noticed you're not as hungry as usual and it's not getting any better.

Symptoms that affect your voice and breathing

Croaky voice or hoarseness

Having a croaky voice or feeling hoarse can be common with colds. But a croaky voice that hasn't gone away on its own should be checked out.

Persistent cough

Coughs are common with colds and some other health conditions. But if an unexplained cough doesn't go away in a few weeks or gets worse, it could be a sign of cancer.

Breathlessness

It's not unusual to feel out of breath every now and then. But if you notice that you're feeling breathless more than usual or for a lot of the time, tell your doctor.

Changes in your poo or pee

Let your doctor know if you've noticed a change in your bowel habits, have problems peeing, or if there's blood in your pee or poo. A change in bowel habits can include constipation, looser poo or pooing more often. Problems peeing might be needing to go more often or urgently, experiencing pain when peeing, or not being able to go when you need to.

These symptoms can all be caused by conditions other than cancer, but it's best to get them checked out.

Unexplained bleeding or blood

Unexplained bleeding can often be caused by something far less serious than cancer, but you should always report it to your doctor.

This includes blood in your poo or pee, and vomiting or coughing up blood - no matter how much or what colour (it could be red, or a darker colour like brown or black). It also includes any unexplained vaginal bleeding between periods, after sex or after the menopause.

Mouth ulcer or patch that won't heal

It's common to get ulcers (small sores) in the mouth when you're a bit run down – they usually get better in about two weeks. But an ulcer or red or white patch that doesn't heal after 3 weeks should be reported to your doctor or dentist.

Persistent bloating

It's quite common to experience a bloated or swollen tummy that comes and goes from time to time. But if you feel bloated most days, even if it comes and goes, talk to your doctor.

Unusual breast changes

Lumps are not the only breast changes to tell the doctor about. Also look out for any change in the size, shape or feel of a breast, or any skin changes, redness, or pain in the breast. And don't forget any nipple changes, including fluid, which could be blood stained, leaking from the nipple if you're not pregnant or breastfeeding.

Breast cancer is most common in women, but whatever your gender it's important to tell your doctor about any unusual breast changes.

30 October 2020

Feeling bunged up? Don't let poo be a taboo

By Katie Powell

Poor bowel health can be debilitating, so educating and getting people talking about their bowel habits is vital. A reported one in five people are too embarrassed to even talk to their GP about constipation, confirming that poo chat can be a taboo subject for many. Opening your bowels is a normal bodily function and something that each and every one of us does - so let's chat about constipation.

What is constipation?

Constipation is a well-known term - however research found that one in five people believe that constipation is when you open your bowels less than once a day. The general consensus however (and included as part of the Rome IV Diagnostic Criteria for Constipation) is that it is defined as:

- Having a poo less than three times a week
- Straining or being in pain when you have a poo
- When poo is often large and dry, hard or lumpy

The Bristol Stool Chart is also a useful diagnostic tool. It is widely used across healthcare settings and can help patients communicate their stool type to their healthcare professional. Type 1 and type 2 on the Bristol Stool Chart indicate constipation.

Bristol stool chart

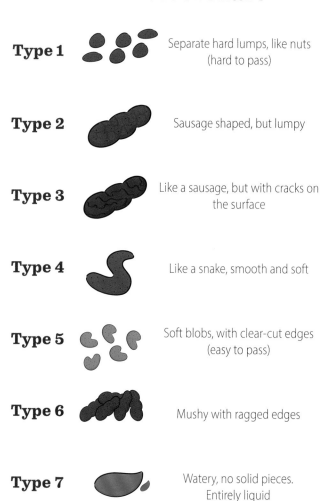

Type 1 — Separate hard lumps, like nuts (hard to pass)

Type 2 — Sausage shaped, but lumpy

Type 3 — Like a sausage, but with cracks on the surface

Type 4 — Like a snake, smooth and soft

Type 5 — Soft blobs, with clear-cut edges (easy to pass)

Type 6 — Mushy with ragged edges

Type 7 — Watery, no solid pieces. Entirely liquid

Constipation - facts and figures

Constipation is one of the most common digestive problems affecting the UK population - so much so that it is estimated that one in seven adults and one in three children are constipated at any one time.

Women are twice as likely to suffer from constipation; pelvic floor disorders are often a cause, as well as pregnancy, due to a change in hormones. It is also well recognised that the older you get, the more likely you are to be prone to constipation - approximately 26% of men and 34% of women over the age of 65 years suffer.

In 2018-19, 76,929 people were admitted to hospital in England with constipation and a whopping £168 million was spent by NHS England treating it.

Not only is it a huge financial burden but for those suffering with the condition, their quality of life can be hugely impacted - 40% of patients with constipation experience an anxiety disorder and 38% experience depression.

How can you improve constipation?

Laxatives are a well-known effective treatment and like all medications, they have a time and a place but should not be seen as a 'quick fix'. Constipation can be effectively treated for most people through diet and lifestyle changes.

Fibre

Often known as the 'roughage' in your diet. Fibres are plant-based carbohydrates which, unlike other nutrients, are not digested in the small intestine and therefore reach the large intestine undigested. Fibre works by bulking out stools, improving your 'transit time' and making stools softer and therefore easier to pass through the digestive system.

In the UK, we are recommended to eat 30g of fibre a day - however on average consumption is much less, at approximately 18g per day. Increasing your fibre intake is likely to help improve constipation - it is important that you make changes gradually, as increasing fibre too quickly may cause bloating or excess wind. Here are some simple suggestions for increasing your fibre intake:

- Swap to a high fibre breakfast cereal such as oats, wholewheat biscuits or bran flakes.
- Choose high fibre snacks such as a portion of fruit, a handful of nuts, oat biscuits or vegetable sticks with hummus.
- Swap to wholegrain carbohydrates such as wholewheat pasta, brown rice, wholewheat noodles and wholewheat or seeded bread.
- Add beans and pulses to your main meals such as minced meat dishes, curries or salads.
- Aim for at least one third, but try for one half, of your plate to be made up of vegetables and/or salad.

Fluid

Keeping yourself hydrated is vital for overall good health - and your hydration status also impacts your bowels. When

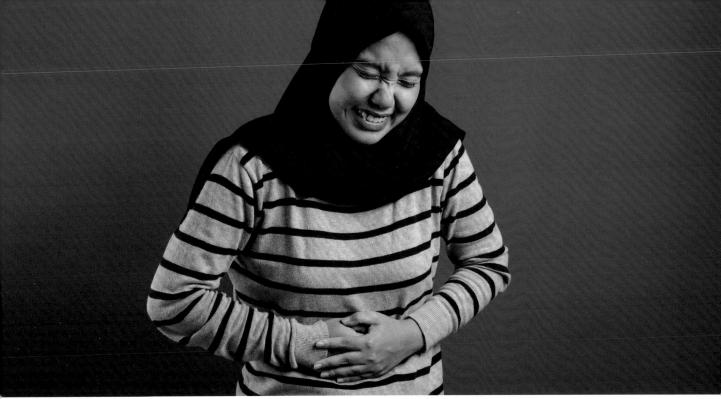

you are dehydrated, the body draws out water from your stools in your large intestine to use elsewhere in the body - this can cause your stools to become dry, hard and lumpy.

The typical adult needs 1.5-2L of fluid a day, or six to eight mugs. A quick, easy way of checking your hydration status is by looking at your urine - it should be clear or a light straw colour. If you are well hydrated already, there is no evidence to suggest that increasing your fluid intake further will help prevent constipation.

All fluids except for alcohol will count towards your fluid recommendation. However, it is important to remember other considerations for some fluids. For example, the impact of high caffeine intake from tea and coffee, particularly for pregnant women, and that fizzy drinks or fruit juices contain high amounts of sugar.

Physical activity

Physical activity is also helpful in improving constipation. Peristalsis is the wave of muscle contractions within the gut. Peristalsis increases with physical activity and therefore can help to speed up the gut transit time and limit the amount of water that is re-absorbed from the stool in the large intestine.

The UK Government recommends that we should aim to do 150 minutes of moderate aerobic activity or 75 minutes of vigorous activity a week. Moderate activity includes brisk walking, dancing, water aerobics or pushing a lawnmower. Vigorous activity includes jogging, fast swimming, football, netball and gymnastics. For some people, these recommendations are not achievable but even a short walk is likely to provide some benefit.

Toilet routine

Toilet routine is just as important as other dietary and lifestyle changes and can make a real difference in improving constipation. Here are some simple tips for improving your toilet routine:

- Aim to have a regular, unhurried routine when opening your bowels. It is important that you give yourself enough time to ensure your bowels are fully emptied.

- If you feel the urge to poo, do not ignore this. The longer your stools stay in your large intestine, the more likely they will become hard and lumpy - and therefore more difficult to pass.

- When you are sat in a 90 degree sitting position (a typical sitting position on a toilet), your bowel is 'pinched', making it more difficult to have a bowel movement. By sitting so that your knees are above your hips, leaning forward with your forearms on your thighs, bulging out your abdomen and straightening your spine, this will 'straighten out' your bowel and will make it easier for you to open your bowels.

Can a dietitian help with constipation?

A dietitian is qualified to provide dietary and lifestyle advice for a range of clinical conditions, including constipation. They are trained to translate the most up-to-date scientific evidence into practical advice for people.

They are likely to ask about your history including past medical history and investigations, medication history, social history, anthropometrics (weight, height, weight loss, etc), any relevant clinical information such as bowel habits and symptoms, and your dietary and lifestyle habits. Based on the information provided, your dietitian will work with you as an individual to create a patient-centred plan that is specific to suit you.

If you feel it would be beneficial for you to see a dietitian, either speak to your GP and ask them to refer to your local NHS Nutrition & Dietetics department or head to the British Dietetic Association Freelance Dietitians webpage to find a dietitian who will be able to see you privately.

Acne: am I cleaning my face enough?

By: Dr Moumita Chattopadhyay

While it's very common in teenagers, acne is a troubling condition for some adults too. Our natural reaction when we see large, inflamed spots appearing on our face is to vigorously clean the area and start applying creams, face masks and anything we can find to reduce the swelling. But is this over-cleaning doing more harm than good? And how often should I be washing my face?

Dr Moumita Chattopadhyay is a leading consultant dermatologist based in Birmingham who specialises in treating adults with acne. In this article, she explains the main causes of acne, how our cleaning habits might be exacerbating it and whether make-up can, in fact, make acne worse.

Why do some adults have acne?

There are several causes of acne in adults. In our skin, we have structures called hair follicles that have tiny sebaceous glands attached to them. These glands produce sebum (oil), which lubricates our hairs. If the glands produce too much sebum, it mixes with dead skin cells and clogs the follicles. This results in inflammation, whiteheads and blackheads on the surface of the skin.

Acne in women

Acne affects women much more than men, mainly due to their fluctuating hormone levels - a lot happens along a woman's hormonal journey. Women might typically see an increase in acne during these times:

- Just before menstruation
- While taking contraception
- During the first few months of pregnancy
- Menopause

These periods of a woman's life can stimulate the sebaceous glands to produce more sebum on the skin surface, and as we mentioned earlier, it can mix with dead cells and go into the hair ducts blocking the pores through which hair comes out. So there is nowhere for the sebum to escape, it builds up, irritates the skin and starts an inflammatory process resulting in red, enlarged spots, whiteheads and blackheads.

What else can trigger acne?

There are many possible triggers for acne flare-ups, such as:

- Certain diseases — polycystic ovarian disease is a condition that can affect women and cause imbalances in their hormones. Unfortunately, this can result in acne flare-ups
- Various medications — lithium is a drug to help treat depression and bipolar disorder which is known to cause spots. Also, steroid medications can trigger acne and this is particularly seen in male bodybuilders
- Genetics — your family history can mean you are more prone to developing acne
- Obese people — Hormones are raised in people who are very overweight and this is a risk factor for acne

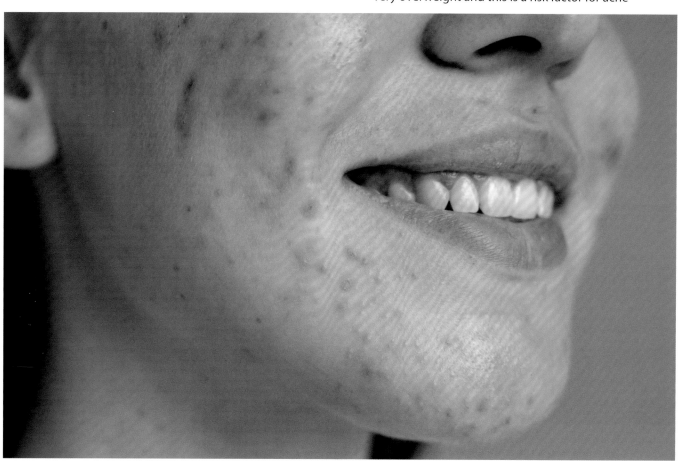

- Smoking — studies show that smoking increases the sebum production in your skin

How is teenage and adult acne different?

While teenagers go through their own hormonal changes, a similar process does occur. The difference is spots will typically appear along the T-zone of the face in teenagers, which is where there is a maximum concentration of these sebaceous glands. Whereas in adults, they will find acne forming along the chin, jawline and neck.

Should I stop wearing makeup if I have acne?

No. You can wear makeup but just be cautious about the kind of makeup you put on your face. It shouldn't be heavy, and you definitely shouldn't be applying thick layers as this will only clog up your pores. Stick to gentle, matte finish and mineral powder-based products.

Oil-absorbing primers can also help; just don't apply anything greasy to your face as you need to allow your hair follicles to breathe. If your skin is already producing a lot of oil, then the hair follicles are already struggling through the layer of sebum and bacteria, so adding more oily-based substances on top of this isn't helping.

One important thing is you **MUST** remove your make-up before going to bed.

While we are sleeping our cells are renewing themselves; dead skins fall off and new cells form. This is the body's **natural exfoliation process** and if you sleep with make-up on your skin, you aren't letting the cells renew, and you'll end up with dead skin, bacteria and make-up clogging up your pores.

To remove your make-up, I recommend lightly wiping your face with a very gentle skin cleanser, but be sure not to scrub your face. You can use gentle wipes if you have to, but nothing with a fragrance and definitely not alcohol-based.

Make sure you check the ingredients in the make-up products and cleaners before buying them. Always buy natural, gentle, water-based and light products that allow your skin to breathe.

What tips do you recommend for people with acne?

Although it is tempting, squeezing your spots and blackheads and exfoliating too much is bad. By doing this, you are pushing bacteria deeper into the skin and irritating it further. Not only does squeezing inflamed spots increase inflammation, but it can also leave permanent scars on your face too - so it's best to leave them to naturally heal.

Additionally, maintaining hygienic and healthy habits is recommended. Wash your face gently with lukewarm water, but no more than twice a day. Washing it more can dry the skin and cause more sebum production.

Do not add anything to your skin that might irritate it; so no harsh facial cleansers or scrubs. For dry skin, it's ok to put on a light moisturiser.

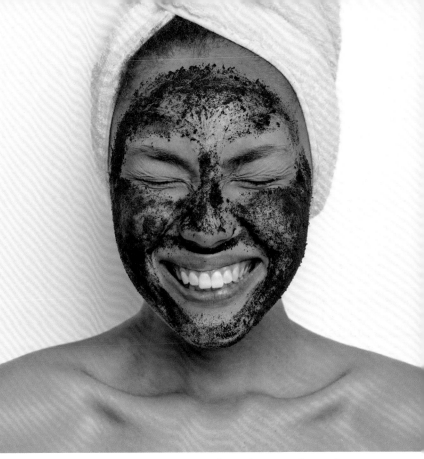

Does acne mean I'm not keeping my face clean enough?

It is not solely related to not keeping the skin clean. While we should remove the dirt and make-up from our faces, the pathology really lies beneath the skin: Acne is driven by a combination of hormones, excess sebum, bacteria, microbiomes of your skin (skin flora), etc. So it hasn't got that much to do with cleanliness.

In addition, the process of inflammation that is going on beneath the skin is what contributes to the acne, rather than an infection occurring from not keeping your face clean.

The bottom line

- Let your skin breathe
- Do not wash your face more than twice a day, use lukewarm water, extremes of temperature irritate the skin
- Scrubbing and vigorously cleaning can make your acne worse
- Use gentle face cleansers, light water-based make-ups
- Never squeeze blackheads or whiteheads
- Always remove your make-up before going to bed
- Limit the use of exfoliation products

28 May 2020

www.topdoctors.co.uk

Teens' teeth

Why is a healthy smile important?

An attractive and healthy smile is important when meeting people and making friends. And it can boost your confidence and help you feel good about yourself.

If you don't look after your teeth and gums properly you could suffer from a number of different conditions that will make you stand out from the crowd for all the wrong reasons:

- Bad breath
- Stained teeth
- Tooth decay
- Gum disease
- Tooth loss
- Dental erosion

Why is a healthy diet important for my oral health?

Every time you eat or drink anything sugary, your teeth are under acid attack for up to one hour. This is because the sugar reacts with the bacteria in plaque and produces harmful acids. Plaque is a build-up of bacteria which forms on your teeth.

It is better to have three or four meals a day rather than lots of snacks.

What is dental erosion?

Dental erosion is the gradual loss of tooth enamel caused by acid attacks. Enamel is the hard, protective coating of the tooth. If it is worn away, the dentine underneath is exposed and your teeth can look discoloured and become sensitive.

Drink up

Acidic foods and drinks and fizzy drinks cause dental erosion.

Still water and milk are the best things to drink. Tea without sugar is also good for teeth as it contains fluoride.

Drink fruit juice just at mealtimes. If you want to drink fruit juices between meals, try diluting them with water.

Snacks

Avoid sugary snacks. If you need to eat between meals try these foods instead:

- Plain popcorn.
- Nuts.
- Cheese.
- Breadsticks.
- Plain yogurt.
- Rice cakes.
- Unsweetened cereal.
- Plain bagels.
- Fresh soup.
- Raw vegetable pieces.
- Fresh fruit.

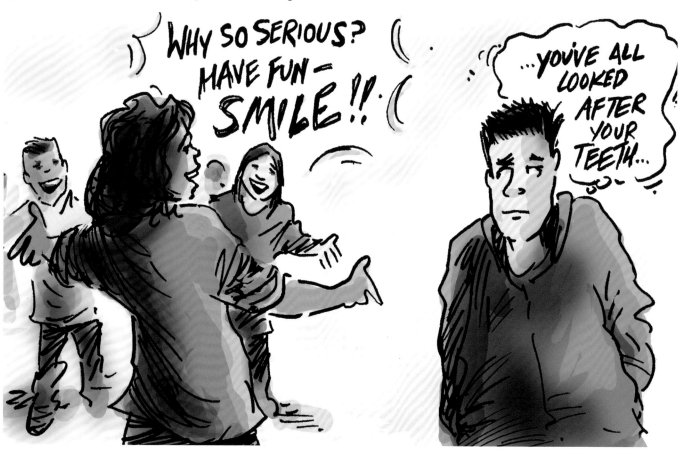

What effects will smoking, alcohol or taking drugs have on my oral health?

Smoking can cause tooth staining, gum disease, tooth loss and - more seriously - mouth cancer. Smoking is also one of the main causes of bad breath.

Alcoholic drinks can also cause mouth cancer. If you smoke and drink you are more at risk.

Alcohol can also increase the risk of tooth decay and erosion. Some alcoholic drinks have a lot of sugar in them, and some mixed drinks may contain acids. So they can cause decay or dental erosion if you drink them often and in large amounts.

Illegal drugs can lead to a range of health problems. Smoking cannabis can have the same effects as smoking tobacco. Other drugs can cause a dry mouth and increase the risk of erosion, decay, gum disease and bad breath. Drugs can also cause you to grind your teeth, which can cause headaches and other problems. Many drugs can cause a craving for sugar, such as sweets and fizzy drinks, which can cause tooth decay.

The human papillomavirus (HPV) is the main cause of cervical cancer and affects the skin that lines the moist areas of the body (such as the mouth). It can be spread through oral sex. Practising safe sex and limiting the number of partners you have may help reduce your chances of getting HPV.

You may hear about teenage girls being offered the HPV vaccine to help prevent the virus. Talk to someone at your medical practice, or your parents or guardians, if you want to know more about this.

Your dentist may ask you questions about your lifestyle choices and general health because these may affect the health of your mouth.

How do I look?

Some people are unhappy with how their teeth look and feel self-conscious smiling in photos or in social situations. But you can have treatment to correct any problems.

How can I improve my smile?

An orthodontic appliance ('brace') will straighten or move your teeth to improve their appearance and the way they work. It can also help to improve the long-term health of your teeth, gums and jaw joints by spreading the biting pressure over all the teeth.

There are many different types of brace and your dental team or orthodontist will be able to talk to you about what is best for you.

Many people want to have whiter teeth. The only person who can whiten your teeth legally for you is a dentist, although there are 'home whitening kits' you can buy, you need to be over 18 to purchase these.

How long will I need to wear a brace?

It depends on how severe the problem is, and it may take anything from a few months to two-and-a-half years. However, most people can be treated in one to two years.

What is tooth jewellery?

Tooth jewellery involves sticking small jewels onto the teeth using dental cement. They should be fitted by a dentist, who can also easily remove them if necessary.

It is important to keep the area around the jewel clean, as plaque can easily build up around it and you will be more likely to get tooth decay.

What are the dangers of mouth piercing?

- Infection.
- The surrounding tissues can become inflamed.
- Blood infections.
- The tongue can swell.
- Teeth can chip and break.
- It can be difficult to talk, eat and swallow.
- It is difficult to keep your mouth clean.
- Dental treatment can be difficult.

How can I protect my teeth when playing sports?

A mouthguard will help protect you against broken and damaged teeth, and even a broken or dislocated jaw.

It is important to wear a professionally made mouthguard whenever you play any sport that involves contact or moving objects.

Ask your dental team about a mouthguard. It is a small price to pay for peace of mind.

Top tips for teens

- Brush your teeth last thing at night and at least one other time during the day. Use a toothbrush with a small- to medium-sized brush head with soft to medium bristles, and brush for two minutes.
- You should use a pea-sized amount of toothpaste that contains 1350ppm to 1500ppm fluoride.
- Have sugary food and drinks just at mealtimes.
- Visit your dental team at least once a year, or as often as they recommend.
- Clean in between your teeth with 'interdental' brushes or floss at least once a day, to help remove plaque and food from between your teeth.
- Use a mouthwash to freshen your breath and kill bacteria.
- Use a straw if you have fizzy drinks, as this helps the drink to go to the back of your mouth and reduces the number of acid attacks on your teeth.
- Wait for at least one hour after eating or drinking anything acidic before you brush your teeth.
- Chew sugar-free gum after eating to help make more saliva and cancel out the acids which form in your mouth after eating.

The above information is reprinted with kind permission from the Oral Health Foundation.
© 2021 Oral Health Foundation

www.dentalhealth.org

Braces and orthodontics

Around a third of children need orthodontic treatment. Find answers to some common questions about braces and orthodontics.

Why have braces?

The purpose of orthodontic treatment is to make the best of your teeth.

This includes straightening your teeth so you're able to care for your teeth and gums more easily, and improving your bite so you can eat more comfortably. And your smile will benefit, too.

Treatment almost always involves using braces to straighten crooked, crowded or protruding teeth, close gaps between teeth, and correct the bite so the top and bottom teeth meet when the mouth is closed.

You'll need to have healthy teeth and gums before you can have a brace fitted.

This is because you must be able to keep your teeth and your brace very clean while you're wearing it to avoid getting tooth decay or gum disease.

Treatment usually lasts from 18 months to 2 years, and visits to the orthodontist are needed every 6 to 8 weeks.

Are braces available on the NHS?

Orthodontic treatment is available on the NHS for young people under the age of 18 at no cost.

NHS orthodontic treatment isn't usually available for adults, but may be approved on a case-by-case basis if needed for health reasons.

Your dentist can give you more information.

What's the best age to have braces?

The ideal age to have braces is usually around 12 or 13, while a child's mouth and jaws are still growing.

The opportunity for improvement in an adult is more limited and treatment is likely to take longer.

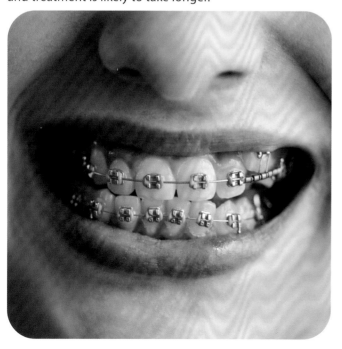

How do I get braces fitted?

Many children don't require a brace, but those who do need to be referred to an orthodontist by their dentist.

By law, only registered specialists can call themselves a specialist orthodontist.

Other dentists may have done extra training so they can also do orthodontic treatment.

Some orthodontists work with orthodontic therapists who can adjust braces under the orthodontist's supervision.

You can look at the specialist list held by the General Dental Council to check an orthodontist's qualifications.

What are braces like?

There are many different types of brace. Some are fixed and stay in all the time. These are the standard brace for NHS treatment in under-18s.

NHS braces are made of metal, but clear ceramic braces, which are less visible, are also available privately.

Removable aligners (thin, clear, flexible plastic mouthguards) may also be available privately.

These fit closely over the teeth and are taken out at mealtimes or to clean them, but are otherwise worn all the time.

How successful are braces?

Orthodontic treatment usually works very well, but you need to stick with it for it to be successful.

You'll need to wear a retainer for some time after your treatment has finished to stop your teeth moving back to the position they were in before treatment.

There are many different types of retainers, which can be either removable or fixed onto the teeth.

Braces can trap food and cause more plaque to build up than usual, so you'll need to take extra care with cleaning your teeth.

You also need to watch what you eat – for example, avoiding sugary foods and drinks.

You should continue to see your regular dentist while having orthodontic treatment.

Can I have private treatment?

Private treatment is widely available. Fees for private orthodontic treatment are usually around £2,500, but can be much higher.

2 November 2018

www.nhs.uk

7 Puberty changes only boys experience

Testosterone is the main hormone responsible for the changes in boys.

It's completely normal for you to experience puberty at any point between the ages of 8 and 14, and these are some of the changes you may notice.

1. Shoulders get wider

Your body is filling out and changing shape during puberty, so you'll notice your shoulders become wider.

2. Muscles get bigger and stronger

Your muscle mass is also building during puberty, so you'll notice your muscles grow and strength improve, particularly your upper body strength.

3. Voice starts to change

Your voice will 'break' as you go through puberty and will become permanently deeper.

During this process, you might find that your voice is very deep one minute and then goes very high the next. This is completely normal.

4. Penis and testicles gets larger

Your penis and testicles will grow in size during puberty, and your scrotum will gradually become darker in colour.

5. You may start to get erections

This is when your penis goes hard and stiff – and can happen at any time.

6. Testicles start to produce sperm

Semen, which is made up of sperm and other bodily fluids, might be released when you have an erection.

This is called ejaculation. Once sperm is made and ejaculation happens, if you had sex without protection you could get someone pregnant.

7. You might have 'wet dreams'

This is when you ejaculate and release semen in your sleep. This is a completely normal part of puberty.

4 Puberty changes only girls experience

Oestrogen and progesterone are the two main hormones responsible for the changes in girls.

Here are some of the changes you can expect to experience as you go through puberty.

1. Hips widen

As your body grows, your hips widen in preparation for you to carry a baby in the future.

2. Breasts start to grow

The oestrogen your body is producing causes your breasts to grow. You might feel itchy or uncomfortable when this happens, but it's completely normal.

3. Changes in your vagina

Your vagina and vulva will grow bigger, and you'll start to produce a clear or white liquid (vaginal discharge) – this is normal and is how your vagina keeps clean and healthy.

If the discharge is yellow, smells or your vagina feels itchy, you should see your doctor as you might have an infection. If you notice more discharge, it might be a sign that your period is going to start soon.

4. Periods (menstruation)

Your periods will start at some point during puberty. You might get period pains in the lead-up to your period and during it too.

Period pains can usually be treated at home, and you shouldn't need to take time off school. Having a warm bath or shower, or placing a covered hot water bottle on your tummy, can also help.

You may not feel like exercising when you have period pains, but gentle exercise can actually help, so maybe try going for a walk.

The above information is reprinted with kind permission from the NHS.
© Crown copyright 2021

www.healthforteens.co.uk

Stages of puberty: what happens to boys and girls

Puberty is when a child's body begins to develop and change as they become an adult.

Girls develop breasts and start their periods. Boys develop a deeper voice and facial hair will start to appear.

The average age for girls to begin puberty is 11, while for boys the average age is 12.

But it's different for everyone, so don't worry if your child reaches puberty before or after their friends.

It's completely normal for puberty to begin at any point from the ages of 8 to 14. The process can take up to 4 years.

Late or early puberty

Children who begin puberty either very early (before the age of 8) or very late (after 14) should see a doctor just to make sure they're in good health.

First signs of puberty in girls

The first sign of puberty in girls is usually that their breasts begin to develop.

It's normal for breast buds to sometimes be very tender or for one breast to start to develop several months before the other one.

Pubic hair also starts to grow, and some girls may notice more hair on their legs and arms.

Later signs of puberty in girls

After a year or so of puberty beginning, and for the next couple of years:

- girls' breasts continue to grow and become fuller
- around two years after beginning puberty, girls usually have their first period
- pubic hair becomes coarser and curlier
- underarm hair begins to grow – some girls also have hair in other parts of their body, such as their top lip, and this is completely normal
- girls start to sweat more
- girls often get acne – a skin condition that shows up as different types of spots, including whiteheads, blackheads and pus-filled spots called pustules
- girls have a white vaginal discharge
- girls go through a growth spurt – from the time their periods start, girls grow 5 to 7.5cm (2 to 3 inches) annually over the next year or two, then reach their adult height
- most girls gain weight (which is normal) as their body shape changes – girls develop more body fat along their upper arms, thighs and upper back; their hips grow rounder and their waist gets narrower

After about 4 years of puberty in girls

- breasts becomes adult-like
- pubic hair has spread to the inner thigh
- genitals should now be fully developed
- girls stop growing taller

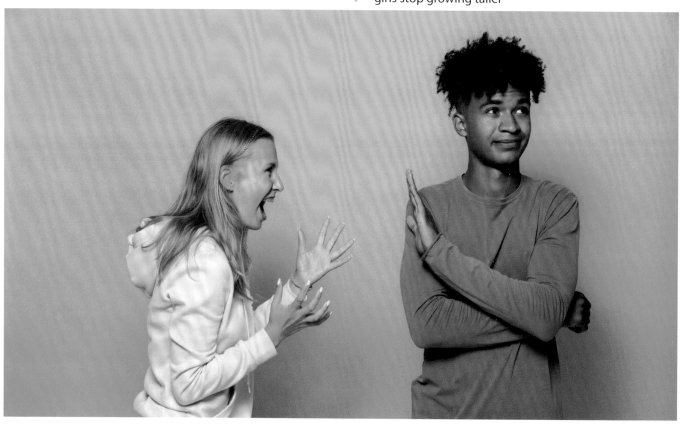

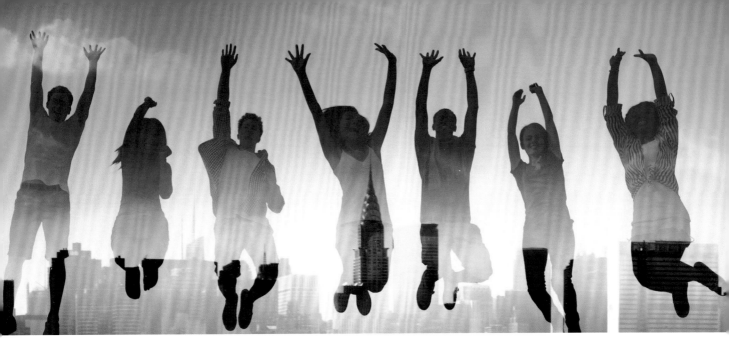

First signs of puberty in boys

- the first sign of puberty in boys is usually that their testicles get bigger and the scrotum begins to thin and redden
- pubic hair also starts to appear at the base of the penis

Later signs of puberty in boys

After a year or so of puberty starting, and for the next couple of years:

- the penis and testicles grow and the scrotum gradually becomes darker
- pubic hair becomes thicker and curlier
- underarm hair starts to grow
- boys start to sweat more
- breasts can swell slightly temporarily – this is normal and not the same as 'man-boobs'
- boys may have 'wet dreams' (involuntary ejaculations of semen as they sleep)
- their voice 'breaks' and gets permanently deeper – for a while, a boy might find his voice goes very deep one minute and very high the next
- boys often develop acne – a skin condition that shows up as different types of spots, including whiteheads, blackheads and pus-filled spots called pustules
- boys go through a growth spurt and become taller by an average of 7 to 8cms, or around 3 inches a year, and more muscular

After about 4 years of puberty in boys

- genitals look like an adult's and pubic hair has spread to the inner thighs
- facial hair begins to grow and boys may start shaving
- boys get taller at a slower rate and stop growing completely at around 16 years of age (but may continue to get more muscular)
- most boys will have reached full adult maturity by the age of 18

Mood changes in puberty

Puberty can be a difficult time for children. They're coping with changes in their body, and possibly acne or body odour as well, at a time when they feel self-conscious.

Puberty can also be an exciting time, as children develop new emotions and feelings.

But the 'emotional rollercoaster' they're on can have psychological and emotional effects, such as:

- unexplained mood swings
- low self-esteem
- aggression
- depression

Puberty support for children

If children are worried or confused about any part of puberty, it may help them to talk to a close friend or relative.

ChildLine's website answers boys' common questions about puberty and girls' common questions about puberty. It also offers free and confidential advice on its telephone helpline, which can be reached on 0800 1111. Children can also look at its puberty message board for girls and puberty message board for boys to see what other young people are asking about.

Puberty support for parents and carers

The Royal College of Psychiatrists website gives advice for parents and carers on what to expect when children hit adolescence, including why they're likely to become sulky, suddenly start dieting, have crushes on friends, and crave excitement.

The FPA (formerly the Family Planning Association) has a range of online leaflets that give advice on talking to your children about growing up, sex and relationships.

16 November 2018

www.nhs.uk

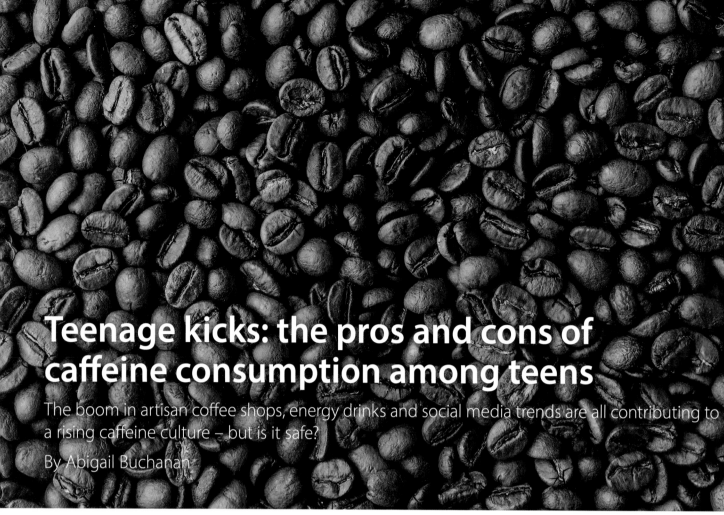

Teenage kicks: the pros and cons of caffeine consumption among teens

The boom in artisan coffee shops, energy drinks and social media trends are all contributing to a rising caffeine culture – but is it safe?

By Abigail Buchanan

I can pinpoint the precise moment my coffee habit started. In my mid-teens, while doing work experience, I would head out to the local coffee shop to do the office tea run and bring what I thought looked like a grown up and sophisticated cappuccino back to my desk. It quickly became a habit and I never looked back. Now in my twenties, I've switched to black Americanos and flat whites and drink around three a day.

I've always focused on the positives of caffeine – it makes me feel more alert and productive – and meeting in coffee shops is one of my favourite ways to socialise. But could developing a taste for thrice-daily flat whites in my teens have done more harm than good?

Caffeine is the most commonly ingested psychoactive substance in the world and coffee the second most popular beverage (after water). It's not harmful in moderation, but evidence suggests the age that people are kickstarting a caffeine habit is getting increasingly younger.

The explosion of coffee culture in the UK, where artisan coffee shops have slowly taken over a dying high street, is surely a factor, as is the rise of cheap, sugar- and caffeine-packed energy drinks. The fact that 'proffee' (a blend of espresso and protein shake) has taken off on TikTok proves that, instead of being associated with tired middle aged office workers drinking a quick pick-me-up, coffee has increasing appeal to young people.

This debate on whether caffeine is safe for children and adolescents is not new – if the old wives' tale is to be believed, coffee stunts a child's growth. That particular claim has been disproved by research, but the question remains: should young people be drinking an addictive substance at all?

The European Food Standards Agency says a daily caffeine intake of up to 3mg per kilogram of body weight 'does not raise safety concerns' for children and adolescents. For the average 14-year-old who weighs 50kg, that translates to 150mg of caffeine. However, a Starbucks flat white contains 130mg of caffeine, an Americano contains 225mg, and one Red Bull contains 80mg – it's easy to see how that guidance could be exceeded without even realising. All it would take is one high street coffee or two caffeinated energy drinks.

Despite coffee's proven health benefits, the negative side effects caffeine consumption can cause are well documented. 'Intakes of caffeine above safe levels can cause anxiety, insomnia, headaches, cardiovascular symptoms and gastrointestinal complaints in some people,' says Helena Gibson-Moore, a nutrition scientist and spokesperson for the British Nutrition Foundation (BNF).

It's clear why many believe young people are more susceptible to caffeine's negative effects. A study cited by the BNF shows that, in the 12-18 age group, daily energy drinks were strongly associated with increased risk of headaches, sleeping problems, irritation and fatigue. New research commissioned by a sports nutrition brand found that almost half of young people aged 18 to 34 struggle with 'chronic lethargy' and 30 per cent experience digestive issues due to caffeinated drinks.

Energy drinks, sales of which increased by 185 per cent between 2006 and 2015, have also been linked to disruptive behaviour in school. An American study notes that caffeine causes a higher incidence of anxiety disorders in adolescents. Plus, according to the BNF, 'the majority of studies that have looked at the health effects of caffeine consumption have been conducted in adults', meaning there is little evidence-based guidance for young people's caffeine consumption.

This paints quite a damning picture. But according to Peter Rogers, professor of biological psychology at the University of Bristol, children and adolescents don't actually react to caffeine in a different way to adults provided they're consuming a safe amount. 'While very little research has been done [on children and the effects of caffeine], a study we published on primary school children found they respond to caffeine much the same as adults do,' he says. 'However, it's possible for young people to drink too much given that some energy drinks contain large amounts of caffeine.'

As with adults, issues arise when young people drink excessive caffeine or use caffeine for the wrong reasons (such as to replace lost sleep). Just as I started to drink coffee on a work experience placement, anecdotal evidence gathered from friends has convinced me that many young people initially start drinking caffeinated drinks to help them work harder or study for exams, which presents a problem in itself.

'I started drinking coffee at 14 because I had dance classes after school, so I had to get up really early to do my homework and wasn't getting enough sleep,' one friend in her twenties tells me. Other daily coffee drinkers tell me they started relying on a caffeine kick to help them study for GCSEs or, more commonly, A-Levels.

When I put this to Rogers, he says: 'Increasing your caffeine intake around the time of exams is not a useful strategy as it could exacerbate anxiety.' The other issue, of course, is that regular caffeine drinkers quickly develop a tolerance to its effects.

While consuming caffeine in moderation may not be actively harmful for young people, there is no evidence to suggest that it has any clear benefits. Plus, as Rogers says, although the negative effects of caffeine don't differ between children and adults, that doesn't change the bottom line: it's a psychoactive substance that can have side effects when consumed in excess. A strong, frothy coffee is undoubtedly my favourite way to start the day – but on reflection, as a teenager, I should have stuck with water.

21 April 2021

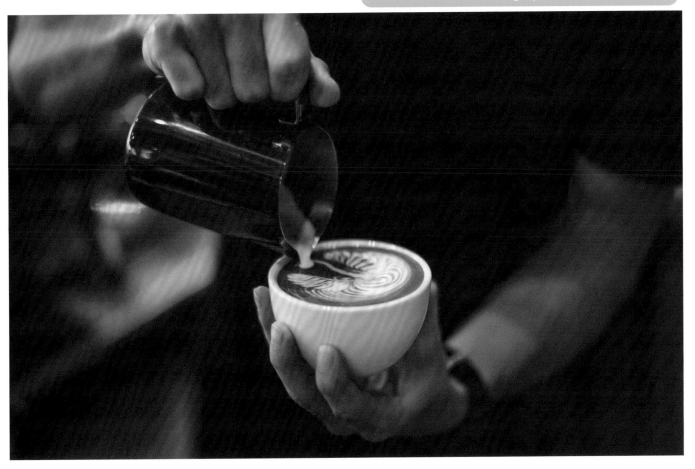

How often should you really shower? Jake Gyllenhaal, Mila Kunis and Kristen Bell spark washing debate

Is there a 'correct' number of times you should be taking a shower? Dermatologists say Jake Gyllenhaal made a good point with his recent comments on bathing being 'less necessary at times'.

By Hollie Richardson

Daily showers are not the done thing in the luxury hills of Hollywood, according to some recent revelations.

The internet was left in a state of shock last week when Jake Gyllenhaal told Vanity Fair that he finds bathing to be 'less necessary at times'. It came after Mila Kunis and Ashton Kutcher said they only bathe their children when they see dirt. And Kristen Bell has admitted she is a 'big fan of waiting for the stink' before washing.

But Dwayne Johnson isn't here for the latest A-list trend. He has jumped into the conversation by telling fans that he is 'the opposite of a "not washing themselves" celeb' and that he in fact takes three showers a day.

Is there really a 'right' number of times to wash per week? Clearly, it's a contentious issue, even away from the Hollywood hills. A 2019 YouGov poll found that nearly half (49 per cent) of its respondents showered once a day, and one in five showered four to six times a week. One in 20 (6 per cent) showered or bathed several times in a day.

'I shower every work day because it makes me feel "ready",' Donna, 38, Edinburgh, tells The Independent. 'I don't feel productive without it. On the weekends, I shower if I'm leaving the house, but I don't bother when I'm not.'

'I work in a hospital and I "need" a morning shower before setting off so that I feel fresh,' says Joe, 34, London. 'On weekends, I'll only get one if I plan to leave the house. But I do feel gross if I don't have one.'

'It's daily shower unless I'm like staying in all day, then I'd just wash my face and have a sink wash,' adds Alice, 30, London. 'Also if I'm extremely hungover, usually on a Saturday, I can't even bring myself to shower.'

Some people go that one step further: 'I get a shower before work and just before bed,' says Carmel, 33, London. 'I've done this since I was a teenager, I just want to always feel "fresh". And during lockdown, I've even added baths during my lunch hour to the routine.'

'I go for a run most days, and I always shower when I get in from one,' adds Tim, 35, Yorkshire. 'A lot of the time, I'll already have had a shower in the morning, which means I quite often have two showers a day.'

The fact that most people want to experience that 'fresh' feeling to help prepare for the day ahead suggests that taking a daily shower is a mental ritual as well as a physical one. A 2008 study reported that participants receiving hydrotherapy for the treatment of depression experienced an improvement after one or two cold showers a day over several weeks.

But is a daily body wash as good for our bodies as it is for our minds?

'From a medical perspective, unless you are visibly dirty or sweaty, you probably don't need to shower more than three times a week,' Dr Sarah Welsh, gynaecology doctor and co-founder at HANX, explains.

'The factors that impact your need to wash include your occupation (if you're doing manual labour or working with patients) and your social and exercise habits. Generally, it's important to especially wash your feet, armpits and groin, as these areas are prone to becoming infected if not kept fresh. And even without Covid, you should ensure you wash your hands regularly.'

But Welsh warns that over washing also had its downsides: 'It can break down the skin's natural barriers and cause soreness and dryness. So, basically, just try to keep it clean on a regular basis.'

Dr Kathy Taghipou, an NHS dermatologist from DermConsult, adds: 'It is recommended to take a shower in the morning as humans tend to perspire at night. Washing in the morning will get rid of sweat and bacteria from the sheets that are sitting on your skin and reduce the chance of infection.'

And Emma Coleman, a dermatology and aesthetics RGN, advises that showering and bathing frequency can be altered according to the seasons: 'It is kinder to the skin to wash on alternate days during the winter, as warm showers and baths can irritate eczema symptoms such as itching, which tend to flare up more during the colder months of the year. But in the summer, you may need to wash your body more frequently due to sweating.'

When it comes to washing your baby, the NHS website states: "You don't need to bathe your baby every day. You may prefer to wash their face, neck, hands and bottom carefully instead. This is often called 'topping and tailing".'

While it's clearly important to wash regularly, it turns out that Gyllenhaal has actually made a pretty valid point about everyday showering being somewhat unnecessary.

9 August 2021

Looking After Your Mind

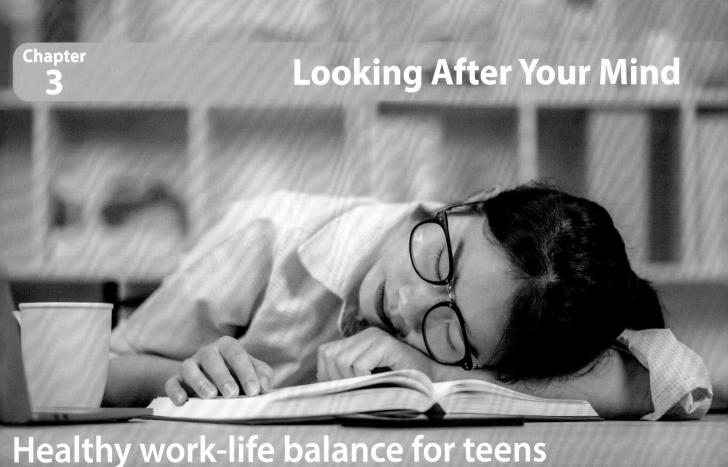

Healthy work-life balance for teens

My mum says it's important to eat healthily and to exercise and to keep a healthy work/life balance so I don't get stressed. I however find this very challenging as there never seems to be enough time in the day to get it all in. Can you please give me some tools to help me with managing my time better so that my life will be more balanced and I can live in a healthier way.

The life of a teenager is very busy and can feel stressful. In this case your mum is 100% right. Eating healthily and learning how to manage your time so that you get enough sleep and exercise are life skills that you will benefit from throughout adulthood. It is far easier to establish good habits and routines when you are young. Good time management can help you find extra time for the things that really matter.

Firstly let me explain why sleep, diet and exercise are so important for your physical and mental health. These 3 factors keep your operating system on top form.

Sleep

There is a very clear link between feeling stressed and lack of sleep. The amygdala is the part of the brain that is the seat of emotions and anxiety. When it senses a threat it goes into fight, flight or freeze mode and when it's tired the brain struggles to tell the difference between threat and non-threat.

During adolescence the natural sleep hormone (melatonin) is released later than in children or adults, which is why teenagers often struggle to fall asleep. Ideally you should be getting 9 hours a night. School starts early so you really need to force yourself to get into bed at a decent time. This can be hard when there's lots of homework and other activities happening.

Be aware that the light from screens delays the release of melatonin, so try switching to a book, music or mindfulness at least an hour before bedtime.

Diet

The gut and the brain are very closely connected and the gut is like our 'second brain'. When the gut is unbalanced it affects your mood and stress levels. Teenagers tend to prefer fast foods but eating healthily (fruit, vegetables and less processed food) will lower stress levels. Don't forget that drinking water also improves your memory and helps you to think clearly. Try to avoid caffeine after 2pm.

Exercise

Any form of physical activity helps you rest and de-stress. It gives you more energy but at the same time improves the quality of your sleep. Even 20 minutes of walking can have a real impact on your well-being, so try to incorporate extra walking into your daily routine, such as getting off 1 bus stop earlier than usual or always committing to walking up escalators and not using lifts.

How can you manage time better?

♦ We often start with very good intentions but after a few days lose momentum. Positive habits are how you create real change, so start small with tiny changes and targets. Getting into the daily routine of doing things in a certain

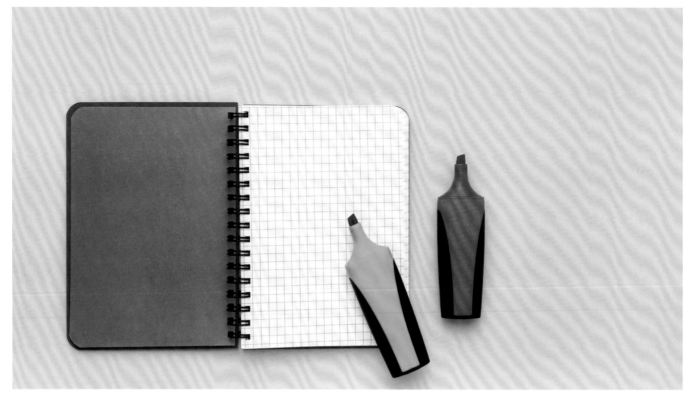

way or order helps you work on auto pilot so you don't have to waste time thinking what to do next.

- Take some time (Sundays are usually best) to think about the coming week and make a list of your goals.

Put these goals into 3 categories:

- What really needs to get done (homework or revision)
- What you would like to get done (less urgent)
- What you want to do (perhaps exercise or seeing friends)

Try to have a real sense of how long each task takes and be a time realist as opposed to time optimist. Your overall productivity will really improve when you begin to understand how long things really take rather than how long you think they will take.

- Use a planner, wall calendar or app to map out your weekly schedule of what you are doing when and how long for. There are so many available but it's about finding one that works for you. Set aside time after school for homework, extracurricular activities, exercise and unstructured down time. Being organised saves a lot of time and stress.

- Set limits on your screen for things like social media or playing games as these activities can steal huge amounts of time without you realising it. Constant screen interruptions strain your brain and contaminate your time. Use a timer in 30 minute intervals for any task, which prevents time passing away without too much thought.

- It's very easy to feel overwhelmed. Break large tasks down into manageable chunks with deadlines and they won't feel as daunting. Small steps make something big seem possible to get the ball rolling and help with procrastination.

- Know yourself and which times of the day you function best. Everyone goes through phases and there are times when you are really in flow and fully focused, times when attention is quite active and times when you are feeling tired. Think about all the tasks you have to do which require full focus and what you can do that's quite easy and repetitive to complete in the time when your attention is flagging, so you can switch tasks and make use of all the different times.

- Chunk your time to minimise constant multitasking and create periods of uninterrupted time to be with friends, family or exercise.

Time management is something that many adults struggle with and needs to be learnt. The best time to start is right now.

It's hard but so valuable to try to spend more time on things that are not urgent but still very important. What matters more than what we are doing is how we feel about it.

Our perception of time is our reality.

Get the best out of your me-time

By Alice Ford

The end of lockdown is almost in sight, but we've still got some time before we get there. So what can you do to make the most of your time right now? We caught up with NCS Grad Alice who gave us her ideas on getting the best out of your me-time...

We all know how easy it is to spend every day of lockdown aimlessly scrolling through social media or binging Netflix shows with a bag of Doritos. And while that isn't the worst way to spend time, it can lead to feeling bogged down, lethargic and even trigger mental health issues.

So, here are my ideas on one person activities you can do to keep yourself busy and feeling inspired! Try to do one or more of these activities every day so that you feel productive, have a routine and have things to look forward to.

Arts and crafts

There are so many crafts to choose from, and with YouTube tutorials you'll be able to find something you love in no time. Why not look up origami, colouring, knitting, embroidery, calligraphy, or more...the list goes on and on!

The world and their mother have decided they're the new Mary Berry right now...and we're here for it! So why not give baking or cooking a go.

A lot of people are doing more online shopping during lockdown, but did you know you can easily revamp the clothes you already have by cropping your old t-shirts, embroidering flowers onto jumpers, or doing some tie-dye.

If you're missing your friends and want to relive your past adventures, you could make a scrapbook or a memory box by collecting your tickets, photographs and postcards and making a collage. Or, make a vision board of all the things you want to do and achieve once all of this is over!

As well as Zoom calls with your friends, try going a bit old school and send them letters. It is really touching to receive handwritten letters in the post!

Using technology positively

While most of the activities so far allow for a nice break from looking at a screen, here are some ways to make the most of the resources online.

Find live streams that you are interested in – such as The Shows Must Go On musical livestreams and National Theatre livestreams if you like theatre! Watching live streams rather than regular videos online helps you have things to look forward to throughout the week.

We all have that one show or film we've been meaning to watch forever but never got around to and now is the perfect opportunity. For me, it's to finally finish the Harry Potter series!

If you like playing games, I suggest The Sims. You log on with the intention of playing for an hour then suddenly it's three hours later and you are still building the same house! It's also a great way to live vicariously through your Sims' non-restricted life right now! Or, if you're looking for something

a bit trickier, play some online escape rooms (or set up your own!).

Skills

It is so important to keep your brain active while you're unable to go to school, university or work, and picking up new skills can help with that.

Why not start a new research project. Find a topic you are interested in and educate yourself; this could be anything from Black Lives Matter to climate change, there are thousands of resources online. (How about taking on the Zooniverse?)

Apps like Duolingo make learning a new language super easy, and will give you something to do every day for a certain amount of time.

If you have an instrument in the house that you haven't touched before, teach yourself to play! Just maybe leave your primary school recorder in the attic...no one wants to hear that!

You could also do things that will keep you active, like digging out your old roller skates or skateboard, doing a 1000 piece puzzle, learning how to juggle or learning how to french braid your hair.

Self-care

Stress levels seem to be high for everyone during lockdown, so it's vital to look after your mental health and your body.

Lockdown is a great opportunity to perfect your skin care routine! Research into your skin type and order some new products that are suitable for you. I find pampering myself with a facemask while watching a movie a great way to relax in the evening.

Another great way to relax and feel more connected with your body is through yoga, meditation or working out. There are thousands of videos on YouTube you can follow. It might feel like a lot of effort once you first start out, but you'll quickly see yourself making progress and begin to enjoy it.

Take a break from screens for a while and do some reading. It stimulates your imagination in a way that TV shows and films do not and it's a great way to detox from technology!

I know lots of people have been rearranging the furniture in their rooms, but how about also setting yourself a challenge to get rid of, or sell, old clothes and items that you no longer need. Being in a tidy room rather than a cluttered one will help you become more productive!

Thank you for reading and remember to look after yourselves and the people around you and know that this restricted lifestyle is not forever.

3 July 2020

Exam stress: 8 tips to cope with exam anxiety

Exam time is really not easy, so you won't be alone in feeling a bit overwhelmed by revision from time to time. But remember: you got this – and these stress-busting tips can hugely help.

By Katie Paterson

Ah, that old familiar knot in your stomach that tells you exams are looming. While some people like to believe a bit of anxiety and pressure can be beneficial around exam time, science suggests otherwise.

When we're stressed, our brains release high levels of cortisol which can cloud the way we think and gets in the way of rational thoughts. Because of this, it's important to stay as cool, calm and collected as you can during the exam period.

Yes, easier said than done.

Follow the practical steps below to relieve exam stress and the awful symptoms. The tips will also improve your productivity, help absorb more information from revision notes, and increase your chances of absolutely smashing it in your exams.

Be sure to take care of yourself ahead of your exams and make time for self-care.

How to reduce exam stress

Here are the best ways to manage your stress levels and stay calm before and during your exams:

Prioritise your time when revising

Prioritising your time, subjects and workload will help reduce your anxiety levels, as you'll be able to ensure that the really important stuff is covered – and at the right time.

If you've got more than one exam to tackle, draw out a simple diagram with dates of each exam and how many topics need covering for each. This will give you a clear idea of how much time you need to dedicate to each exam topic and when you need to get started on your revision, so there won't be any nasty surprises.

As you progress through your revision, tick off the topics that you've completed – this will give you a small sense of achievement, knowing that you've finished something and are making your way to the finish line.

Make a revision timetable

This is pretty closely related to the tip above, but we can't emphasise enough how taking a bit of time to get yourself in order will make you feel more confident for these exams.

As our step-by-step guide to becoming ridiculously organised rightly states, making a revision schedule and writing to-do lists each day will keep you super prepared and on track to getting everything done – and on time.

Working out a daily routine and sticking to it is also good for the soul, as you'll feel a lot more in control of how your day pans out. Remember to factor in regular breaks (we recommend at least 10 minutes every hour and a half or so, if not more) as these will do you wonders.

Exercise and eat healthily

Sometimes the idea of exercising during times of high stress feels like the last thing you want to do, but we guarantee you will feel better afterwards. In fact, you could even have a bit more energy to do an hour more revision afterwards if you're feeling up to it.

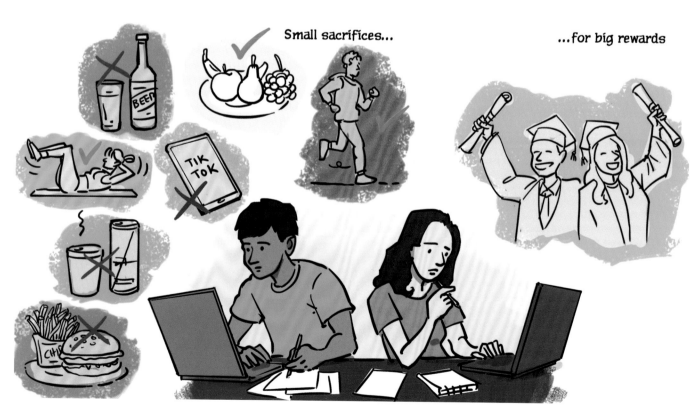

Small sacrifices...

...for big rewards

Exercise gets your blood flowing and your heart pumping. It's a proven stress-buster as it fills your brain with endorphins, which are basically happy hormones. So, once you stop working out, you can feel a lot more alert than you had been earlier.

Give yourself that push to go out for a run, visit the gym, or even just head out for a brisk walk if you fancy a lighter form of exercise.

Eating the right foods during stressful times is also absolutely crucial for mental health and wellbeing.

Take breaks from social media before exams

Stepping away from social media during the exam period, as hard as it might be, will do wonders for your stress levels.

Checking the latest updates on Instagram, Facebook and the like while revising is the worst type of procrastination possible, as we all know how quickly the time disappears when you're swiping through your social feeds.

In addition to this, many of your friends will be in the same boat, so are likely to be talking a lot about how much they're studying (or not studying). This is likely to stress you out even more, or at least influence how much time you're spending revising.

If you need a bit of help unchaining yourself from your phone, give the Hold app a go. Hold gives you real rewards (including Amazon vouchers, cinema tickets and free coffee) for simply avoiding the use of your phone.

You get points every 20 minutes, meaning you can break up your revision periods with some well-earned rests (and well-needed – science says that revision is much less effective if you study for any longer than about 90 minutes straight).

Put your worries into perspective

This is perhaps easier said than done, but try not to give yourself such a hard time. You're doing your best and that's the best you can do! Keep your eye on the bigger picture, and remember that one "meh" result isn't the end of the world.

Putting yourself under a lot of pressure can have a negative effect, and as much of a cliché as this is, worrying really doesn't solve anything.

Being kind to yourself during periods of high anxiety is likely to give you a bit more motivation to work harder, so take a little time out from revision to pamper yourself and catch up with your nearest and dearest.

Cut out caffeine, alcohol and nicotine

We know, we know, cutting out coffee during exam time seems like an impossible task. How are you ever going to stay awake long enough to memorise that 300-page textbook without your good friend caffeine to get you through? Or cigarettes to help you relax afterwards?

Well, caffeine is a stimulant and will increase your stress levels rather than reduce them, and the same applies to nicotine. Avoid drinking more than one cup of coffee a day and cut the cigs if you can. And remember, fewer fags means more savings!

If you can't cut them out completely, try to at least monitor your consumption. You could always try swapping the coffee for herbal tea or water, which will keep your body hydrated and allow you to cope better with stress. Plus, you can swap the ciggies for chewing gum.

This might sound obvious, but try to avoid alcohol during exams periods too. Alcohol can act as a depressant when consumed in large quantities and as a stimulant when consumed in smaller quantities – neither of which is helpful as they can both send your stress levels through the roof.

Cutting out all of these substances will also improve your sleep which, now more than ever, will help you massively.

Do mock exams at home

One of the most common reasons for feeling stressed ahead of exams is not being sure what to expect on the day, such as what questions you're likely to be asked, and how best to approach answering them. The best way to overcome this? Practice – and plenty of it.

If you can, try to find examples of past exam questions for your course to get an idea of what topics have come up in previous years.

Or, if there aren't any past exam questions available, think about what essay/assignment titles you've been set by lecturers throughout the year and think of other questions that are similar to these.

It's particularly helpful to try tackling mock exam questions on topics you're less confident with so that you can prepare plans and practise answering them, in case they do come up in the exam.

By practising how to approach your answers on a range of topics, including your most and least favourite ones, you can put yourself in a great position to show exam markers how much you know and ace even the hardest exam questions.

Improve your exam time management

It's also common for students to worry about time management in exams. If you're concerned about running out of time at the end and leaving questions unfinished, or rushing through questions and finishing the exam too early, practice, again, will massively help with this.

When practising mock exam questions, be strict with yourself over timings so that you don't run over the amount you're allowed in the exam.

In particular, use these practice exams to get yourself organised and work out how long you should leave yourself to plan answers in the exam, and how long you should be spending on each section of your answer.

If, at first, you find yourself unable to finish your answers on time or you have way too much time left over at the end, keep practising until you really nail the timings.

It's worth asking your lecturer to take a look through your practice answers to get an idea of areas that you could improve on, and to see if there are any parts of your argument you could develop further. Some teachers will be more willing to do this than others, but if you never ask, you'll never know.

With all this practice, by the time you reach your exam, you'll be a pro with timings and have a great idea of what kinds of questions to expect on the day. Just in case you didn't believe us before, we hope you do now that you really have got this.

17 June 2020

Self-care on a budget: 10 things to try

Self-care is incredibly important in helping manage and prevent depression.

However, as those of us who struggle with poor mental health are more likely to have financial problems – especially if we are unable to work – there are often real limitations in the amount we can 'budget' to look after ourselves.

But while spa days and shopping sprees are undoubtedly expensive, there are many other acts of self-care that cost very little or are in fact free.

1. Drink up

Being even the tiniest bit dehydrated can have a negative impact on our mood, so ensuring we drink enough water is one of the simplest ways we can look after ourselves. Normal tap water is fine.

If you're not fussed about water, herbal teas (the non-caffeinated kind) also count, and you can pick up boxes relatively inexpensively – especially if you choose own-brand over premium labels. As an added bonus, some herbs (such as chamomile) can soothe symptoms of depression and anxiety. As a few herbs can impact on the efficacy of drugs, do check the information sheet/talk to your doctor if you are on medication.

2. Eat well

We've talked about the benefits of healthy eating before, and contrary to popular belief, eating well doesn't have to be expensive.

Yes goji berries and superfood salads are good for us, but so are baked beans and tinned fish! Our podcast on food and mental health shares several low-cost nutrition ideas, and there are plenty of blogs out there where you can find inspiration: for example *Cooking on a Bootstrap*.

3. Sleep

Getting a good night's sleep is one of the kindest things we can do for ourselves, and better still it's completely free. However, as depression often comes hand-in-hand with sleep problems, we know that can be easier said than done.

You can improve your chances of getting a good night's kip by limiting caffeine after 2pm and implementing a 'bedtime routine' – a series of calming activities you do every night to tell your body and your brain it's time for bed. Limiting screen time in the evenings can also be really helpful, as the light given off by your devices can be disruptive. Our podcast on sleep explains more.

4. Move it

Although it's often the last thing we feel like doing – especially when we're depressed – getting moving is a great way to show ourselves self-care. Exercise has innumerable health benefits, and even a short burst of movement triggers endorphins and gives us that feel good glow.

You don't need a pricey gym membership to exercise either. You can dance in your bedroom to your favourite tunes, follow along with free fitness videos on YouTube, or you can simply pop some trainers on and head out for a walk or run. Exercising outside has additional benefits too.

5. Get out

We love our blanket forts and duvet days (sometimes they are much needed), but we also know how important it is to get outside.

Sunlight and fresh air are instant mood-boosters – and are available to us all, completely free. Research suggests that exposure to natural surroundings is beneficial to physical and psychological wellbeing, so if you can get out into green space (even if it's just your local park) all the better.

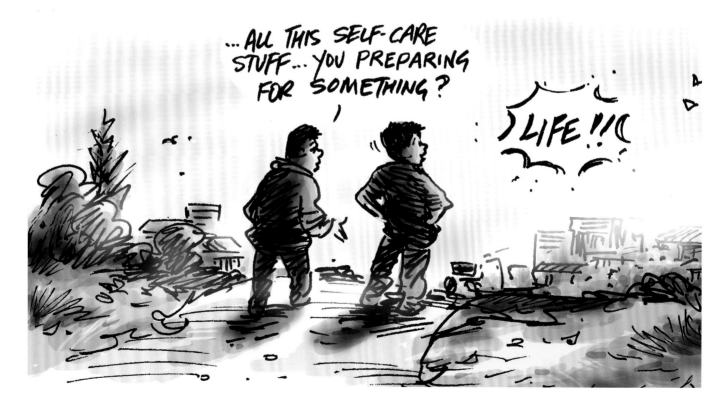

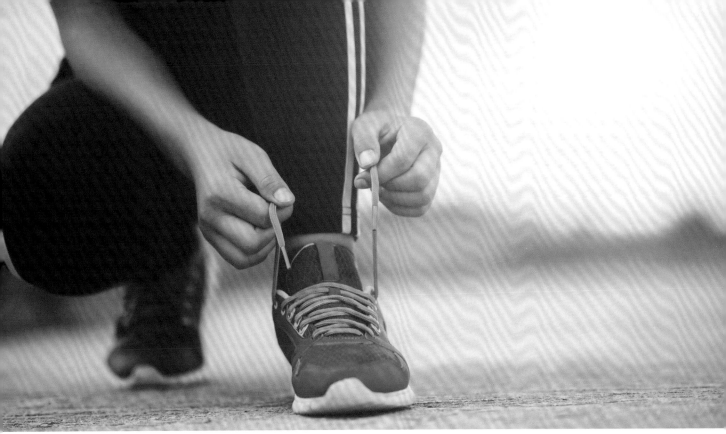

6. Get creative

Engaging in creative activities is a fantastic – and fun – way to integrate self-care into your day, and it needn't be expensive.

We are all innately creative (even those of us who may think otherwise!) and there are so many different ways we can express our creativity. Writing, knitting, sewing, singing, cooking, painting, sculpting, gardening, restoring furniture, playing with make-up, writing computer code... activities like these are beneficial for our wellbeing: they bring us into the present moment, boost feel-good chemicals in our brain, and give us a sense of achievement.

7. Clean up

There is a bit of a trend for decluttering at the moment, and with good reason. The environment in which we live can have a real impact on our mood. If our surroundings stress us out, take up headspace, or make day-to-day living harder than it needs to be, we can definitely benefit from clearing up. (And if we sell any of the stuff that we declutter, our wallets can benefit too!)

As well as decluttering physical items (the contents of our wardrobe, the random drawer of junk in the kitchen, the piles of paper lying about), we can also declutter digitally: think unwanted software that slows the computer down, unread emails or even facebook friends.

8. Treat yourself

While clearing up can be undoubtedly helpful, there *is* something lovely about having new things (that's why we created the BuddyBox!). Of course when we're on a budget, it's not wise to buy stuff willy nilly, but there are ways to get new things on the cheap.

Libraries are a good starting point: if you can't concentrate on books (we struggle to read when we're unwell), there are audio books and DVDs. Plus some local libraries reduce fees for those with disabilities – worth looking into if that applies to you. Then there are charity shops: you'll be surprised by some of the awesome things you can find, and you can treat yourself while helping others. There are also bargains and freebies to be found online: look at sites like freecycle or community Facebook groups.

9. Build boundaries

Those of us who struggle with depression often have issues with low self-esteem, and look externally for approval and validation. If you find yourself regularly putting other people's needs before your own – saying 'yes' when you want to say 'no', exhausting yourself to fulfil other's expectations – you may benefit from working on your boundaries.

You are the most important person in your life (yes, really!), so you need to learn to make your needs a priority. Addressing wonky boundaries can feel like a scary task but you'll feel the benefits almost immediately. And of course looking after yourself in this way doesn't cost financially.

10. Rest up

Many of us have high expectations of ourselves, and feel like we should always be productive: always giving, always doing. Continually putting stress on ourselves in this way is a sure fire road to burnout.

As hard as it might feel sometimes, one of the best things you can do for yourself is STOP. Really. Allow yourself to just be. Run yourself a lovely bath, lie on the floor and stare at the ceiling, watch some nonsense on TV. Letting yourself rest is a fantastic act of self-care, and it doesn't cost a penny.

Over to you

Sharing is caring: please share this article to help others, you never know who might need it.

www.blurtitout.org

Key Facts

- Self-care is a much broader concept which essentially includes the practice of taking an active role in protecting your own wellbeing (emotional, physical, environmental and social), particularly during periods of stress. (page 6)

- 46% of 15 year olds have decay in their permanent teeth. (page 8)

- Over 80% of secondary school pupils in the UK receive teenage vaccinations. (page 8)

- Young people often report turning first to their family for information, help and advice, with the exception of sex and relationships and parental conflict. (page 9)

- The HPV vaccine has led to an 89% reduction in preinvasive cervical disease. (page 10)

- The prevalence of high-risk HPV has reduced with the increasing number of young women who receive the vaccine. (page 10)

- More than a quarter of 15 year olds reported being embarrassed to smile or laugh due to the condition of their teeth. (page 10)

- Measles and mumps cases have nearly doubled in recent years. (page 11)

- If 95% of children receive the MMR vaccine, it's possible to get rid of measles. (page 11)

- Vaccinations prevent up to 3 million deaths worldwide every year. (page 11)

- The main ingredient of any vaccine is a small amount of bacteria, virus or toxin that's been weakened or destroyed in a laboratory first. (page 12)

- In the UK we have one of the most successful immunisation programmes in the world. This means that dangerous diseases, such as polio, diphtheria or tuberculosis, have pretty much disappeared in the UK. (page 13)

- From September 2019, boys aged 12 and 13 in the UK were offered vaccination against the Human Papillomavirus (HPV) for the first time. (page 15)

- HPV types 16 and 18 contribute to 50% of penile cancers, 80% of anal cancers, 20% of mouth, and 30% of throat cancers. (page 15)

- In both the US and the UK, the majority of cancers caused by HPV are not cervical. (page 15)

- There are over 200 different types of cancer. (page 18)

- One in five people are too embarrassed to even talk to their GP about constipation. (page 20)

- One in seven adults and one in three children are constipated at any one time. (page 20)

- In 2018-19, 76,929 people were admitted to hospital in England with constipation and a whopping £168 million was spent by NHS England treating it. (page 20)

- The typical adult needs 1.5-2L of fluid a day, or six to eight mugs. (page 21)

- The UK Government recommends that we should aim to do 150 minutes of moderate aerobic activity or 75 minutes of vigorous activity a week. (page 21)

- Acne affects women much more than men. (page 22)

- The ideal age to have braces is usually around 12 or 13, while a child's mouth and jaws are still growing. (page 26)

- The average age for girls to begin puberty is 11, while for boys the average age is 12. (page 28)

- Caffeine is the most commonly ingested psychoactive substance in the world. (page 30)

- Almost half of young people aged 18 to 34 struggle with 'chronic lethargy' and 30 per cent experience digestive issues due to caffeinated drinks. (page 31)

- Sales of energy drinks increased by 185%t between 2006 and 2015. (page 31)

- 49% of people shower once a day, and one in five showered four to six times a week. (page 32)

- Unless you are visibly dirty or sweaty, you probably don't need to shower more than three times a week. (page 32)

- Teenagers should be getting 9 hours sleep a night. (page 33)

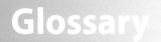

Adolescent

A young person - someone in a transitional phase between child and adult.

Angst

A feeling of anxiety or apprehension.

Anxiety

Feeling nervous, worried or distressed, sometimes to a point where the person feels so overwhelmed that they find everyday life very difficult to handle.

Body image

Body image is the subjective sense we have of our appearance and the experience of our physical embodiment. It is an individual's perception of what they look like or how they should look like. It can be influenced by personal memory along with external sources such as the media and comments made by other people.

Caffeine

Caffeine is a natural stimulant found in drinks like tea, coffee and cola.

Cervical cancer

Cancer that develops in a woman's cervix (the entrance to the womb from the vagina). In its early stages it often has no symptoms. Symptoms can include unusual vaginal bleeding which can occur after sex, in between periods or after menopause. The NHS offers a national screening programme; for all women over 24 years old.

Diet

The variety of food and drink that someone eats on a regular basis. The phrase 'on a diet' is also often used to refer to a period of controlling what one eats while trying to lose weight.

Exam Stress

A feeling of nervousness, fear or worry before or during a test.

Exercise

Physical activity that helps to improve and maintain a healthy body and mind. Exercise can be as easy as walking, swimming or dancing, to more intensive activity such as weight training, aerobics or High-Intensity Interval Training (HIIT).

Fitness

The condition of being physically healthy (e.g. described as being in shape). Remember, fitness can also apply to our mental health and well-being. A high level of fitness is usually the result of regular exercise and a proper nutrition regime.

HPV vaccination

The vaccine is effective at stopping people getting the high-risk types of HPV that cause cancer, including most cervical cancers and some anal, genital, mouth and throat (head and neck) cancers. In England, all boys and girls aged 12 to 13 years are routinely offered the 1st HPV vaccination when they're in Year 8 at school. The 2nd dose is offered 6 to 24 months after the 1st dose. HPV vaccination

Immunisation

Immunisation is the process whereby a person is made immune or resistant to an infectious disease, typically by the administration of a vaccine.

Junk food

`Junk` food is a widely-used term for unhealthy and fatty food with little nutritional value. It is usually associated with `fast` or takeaway food.

Mental health/well-being

Everyone has 'mental health'. It includes our emotional, psychological and social well-being. It affects how we think, feel, and act. It also helps determine how we handle stress, relate to others, and make choices. Mental health is important at every stage of life, from childhood and adolescence through adulthood.

Mindfulness

Mind-body based training that uses meditation, breathing and yoga techniques to help you focus on your thoughts and feelings. Mindfulness helps you manage your thoughts and feelings better, instead of being overwhelmed by them.

Screen time

A term used to refer to the amount of time someone (usually young children) spends in front of a screen. For example, a tablet, smartphone or computer.

Self-esteem

A term referring to how an individual feels about their body. Relating to self-confidence, if a person has low self-esteem they may feel unhappy with the way they look. Alternatively, if a person has good/high self-esteem then they may feel particularly confident about their appearance.

Sugar

Sugar is a carbohydrate that is a naturally-occurring nutrient that makes food taste sweet. There are a number of different sugars: glucose and fructose are found in fruit and vegetables; milk sugar is known as lactose; maltose (malt sugar) is found in malted drinks and beer; and sucrose comes from sugar cane or beet and is often referred to as `table` or `added` sugar. It also occurs naturally in some fruit and vegetables

Vitamins

Organic compounds that are essential to the body, but only in very small quantities. Most of the vitamins and minerals we need are provided through a balanced diet: however, some people choose to take additional vitamin supplements.

Activities

Brainstorming

◆ Brainstorm what you know about teenage health issues.

◆ Make a mindmap of different self-care activities.

◆ Brainstorm what you know about keeping healthy.

Research

◆ Research the levels of physical activity in young people of your age group. How much exercise should they do in a week? Create an exercise plan which could fit into their daily routine. For example, use the stairs instead of a lift, walk instead of taking the bus.

◆ Did you know that caffeine is bad for teenagers' brains? Research food and drinks that contain caffeine and make a graph to show your findings. Pick at least five different foods and drinks.

◆ In small groups, do some research into vaccines. Choose one vaccine and find out as much as you can about it. Produce a poster with some facts and statistics about your chosen vaccine.

◆ Do some research into hygiene. What are the benefits of good hygiene? Make a list of your results.

◆ Research self-care. Create a presentation on different self-care activities that people may enjoy.

◆ Create a questionnaire to see how often people do self-care activities. Ask a wide range of age groups and compare the different activities that people do according to age.

Design

◆ Design a leaflet about mental health in teenagers. It should list the signs of depression or anxiety and give ideas as to how to deal with this condition.

◆ Choose an article from this topic and design an illustration that highlights its key message.

◆ Design an app that will give students tips and advice on how to use self-care to improve themselves.

◆ Choose an article from this book and create an infographic that displays key information.

◆ Create a poster on dental hygiene.

◆ Create a poster with a self-care routine for teens.

◆ Design a poster to promote mindfulness.

◆ Design a leaflet to help teens with hygiene routines.

◆ Create a TikTok or Instagram reel to show some free or low-cost self-care activities.

Oral

◆ Choose an illustration from this topic and, in pairs, discuss what you think the artist was trying to portray with this image. Does the illustration work well with its accompanying article? If not, why not? How would you change it?

◆ Interview your parents, teachers or others who are older than you and find out how healthy they were when they were younger. How much exercise did they do? What were their diets like? Do they feel healthier now? Write some notes and feedback to your class.

◆ As a class, discuss caffeine and the risks that it has to teen health.

◆ In pairs, talk about ways you can use self-care to help your mental health.

Reading/Writing

◆ Read the article 'Sometimes self-care is doing the things you don't want to do' and list some ways that you can protect your own wellbeing.

◆ Write one paragraph of what self-care means to you.

◆ Write a definition of anxiety.

◆ Imagine you are an Agony Aunt/Uncle and you have received a letter from a young boy telling you he is stressed about his forthcoming exams. He is frightened of letting his parents down as they have high expectations of him. He feels like he cannot cope. Write a suitable reply.

◆ Write a blog post imagining you are a teenager who is struggling to sleep.

Acknowledgements

Images

Cover image courtesy of iStock. All other images courtesy of Freepik, Pixabay and Unsplash.

Illustrations

Simon Kneebone: pages 4, 24 & 38. Angelo Madrid: pages 2, 14 & 36.

Additional acknowledgements

Page 16: *About cervical screening* – www.jostrust.org.uk/about-us/how-we-write-our-content/editorial-policy

Page 17: *How do I check for cancer?* – Cancer Research UK, https://www.cancerresearchuk.org/about-cancer/cancer-symptoms/how-do-i-check-for-cancer, Accessed August 2021.

Page 18-19: *Signs and symptoms of cancer* – Cancer Research UK, https://www.cancerresearchuk.org/about-cancer/cancer-symptoms, Accessed August 2021.

With thanks to the Independence team: Shelley Baldry, Danielle Lobban, and Jackie Staines.

Tracy Biram

Cambridge, September 2021